diabetes
eat & enjoy

CHRISTINE ROBERTS
JENNIFER McDONALD
MARGARET COX

THIRD EDITION

NH
NEW
HOLLAND

We dedicate this book to our children:

Christopher, Rebecca, Erica, Ryan, Naomi and Jacqui.

This edition published in the UK in 2001 by
New Holland Publishers (UK) Ltd
London • Cape Town • Sydney • Auckland

Garfield House, 86 Edgware Road, London W2 2EA, United Kingdom
80 McKenzie Street, Cape Town 8001, South Africa
Level 1, Unit 4, 14 Aquatic Drive, Frenchs Forest, NSW 2086, Australia
218 Lake Road, Northcote, Auckland, New Zealand

Published in Australia in 2001 by
New Holland Publishers (Australia) Pty Ltd

First published in 1990
Reprinted 1990 and 1992 (twice)
Revised edition 1995
Reprinted 1996 (twice), 1998, 1999
Third edition 2001

ISBN 1 85974 942 9

Publisher: Averill Chase
Project Editor: Sophie Church
Designer: Nanette Backhouse
Photographer: Ben Dearnley
Stylist: Vicky Liley
Home Economist: Kim Megan Passenger

Consultant Dietician (UK edition): Jill Scott B.Sc. SRD Nutrition and Dietetic Consultant

Printed by Times Offset
Reproduction by Pica, Singapore

All meal plans in this book have been presented as samples only. Anyone wishing to follow
these meal plans should first seek the advice of a qualified dietitian.

Accessories provided by Country Road Homewares, Mud (Australia), Freedom Furniture,
Made In Japan, Mosmania, Shack.

CONTENTS

ACKNOWLEDGEMENTS

There are a number of people who have helped and encouraged us in the writing of this book. We would like, firstly, to acknowledge Diabetes Australia, their Health Care and Education Committee, and their National Marketing Committee, for their support.

We'd especially like to thank Jacqui Roberts for undertaking the difficult task of analysing the recipes and meal plans. The expertise, advice and hard work of René Gordon, our original publisher, and her assistants Joy Bowers, Joslin Guest and Des Carroll have made this book a reality.

Most importantly, we thank our families, and especially our husbands—Noel Roberts, Michael Hall and Jack Cox. Without their support, patience, encouragement and understanding, we could never have completed *Diabetes Eat & Enjoy*.

Christine Roberts, Jennifer McDonald, Margaret Cox
March 2001

ABOUT THE AUTHORS

Christine Roberts A.P.D. is Director of Melbourne Dietetic Centre and Consultant Dietitian to hospitals, commercial organisations and in private practice. She has been involved with diet and diabetes for many years, and has co-authored a number of papers. She was a member of the Working Party for Nutritional Resources, Diabetes Australia in conjunction with the Dietitians Association of Australia, in 1988. She co-authored the successful *Food for Sport Cookbook* and the *Healthy Heart Cookbook* (for the National Heart Foundation). She was also a contributor to Professor Pincus Taft's book, *Diabetes Mellitus*.

Jennifer McDonald A.P.D. is Manager of Nutrition and Dietetics at St Georges Health Service, Melbourne, and consultant to a number of other organisations. She has been involved in writing many publications for people with diabetes and was a member of the Working Party for Nutrition Resources, Diabetes Australia in conjunction with the Dietitians Association of Australia, in 1988. She has co-authored a number of scientific papers dealing with diet and diabetes, in association with other top researchers in the field.

Margaret Cox A.P.D. has been involved in both research and clinical work with people with diabetes for many years. For three years she was nutrition co-ordinator at the International Diabetes Institute, one of Australia's leading diabetes research and educational organisations, and was involved in the development of diabetes education programs and educational resources for people with diabetes. She co-authored the *Healthy Heart Cookbook* for the National Heart Foundation.

INTRODUCTION

As dietitians working with people with diabetes, we are constantly being asked to provide individuals with all the information they need about diet, cooking and eating. In the course of our work over the years, we were very aware how little simple, straightforward and up-to-date information there was about the relationship between food and diabetes. Many people with diabetes don't have enough detailed, yet easily understood, information about the way in which the food they eat affects their control of diabetes, and this makes them unsure of how to plan or prepare their meals.

In the past few years, there have been major changes in the principles of eating for people with diabetes. Where in the past people with diabetes were treated as being different, today we realise that the ideal diet for everyone is perfect for people with diabetes too.

Clearly, there was a need for a book that explained in simple terms the relationship between diabetes and food, laid out the guidelines needed for good management today, and included delicious and healthy recipes ideal for everyone, not just those with diabetes.

Diabetes Eat & Enjoy does just that. Through this book we hope that you will have more confidence in your ability to maintain good health and enjoy the pleasures of the table.

SO WHO HAS DIABETES?

More and more people are being diagnosed with diabetes, so it is difficult to give accurate information about the number of people with diabetes in the UK. However, it is estimated that approximately 1.4 million people have diabetes. This figure is projected to double by the year 2010.

WHERE TO GO FOR FURTHER HELP

- The starting point should be your local GP practice: here you will find access to a number of services to help you manage your diabetes.
- Your doctor will be able to refer you to a State Registered dietician who is likely to be based at the local hospital.
- For more information about State Registered Dieticians contact:
  The British Diabetic Association
  5th Floor, Elizabeth House
  22 Suffolk Street
  Queensway
  Birmingham B1 1LS.

Diabetes UK (formerly the British Diabetic Association)

Diabetes UK is the largest UK charity devoted to the care and treatment of diabetes. It is also one of the largest funders of diabetes research.

Diabetes UK is committed to providing education and support to people with diabetes. They provide:

- a careline (tel: 020 7636 6112)
- books
- magazines
- booklets

They also provide support for healthcare professionals working with people with diabetes. Diabetes UK can be contacted at:

10, Queen Anne Street
London W1M 0BD
Tel: 020 7323 1531
Email: info@diabetes.org.uk
Website: www.diabetes.org.uk

NOTE: The information in this book is current at the time of publication. Research into diabetes continues and areas of management may undergo further change.

KNOWLEDGE IS SWEET

Diabetes mellitus is not new. It may be as old as humanity. Certainly, it has been with us throughout recorded history, but only in 1921 did we learn to treat it with some effectiveness, and only in the past twenty years have we devised a new way of eating for people with diabetes. Over the past eighty or so years, diabetes has changed from being a life-threatening condition to one that requires a change of lifestyle and, where necessary, medication.

WHAT IS DIABETES?

You need to know what diabetes is before you can take an active part in managing your own health care.

'Diabetes' comes from the ancient Greek word for 'siphon', referring to the large amount of sugar-containing urine passed by people with uncontrolled diabetes, and 'mellitus' for the characteristic sweet taste of the urine. Diabetes (more accurately diabetes mellitus) is simply too much sugar in the blood. This sugar is in the form of glucose. Diabetes occurs when the system which controls the amount of glucose in the blood no longer works properly.

But where does it all begin? Everyone has glucose in their blood all the time. It provides energy (or fuel) to keep the body working, much like the petrol in a car.

Where does glucose come from?

Glucose comes from the food we eat. When we eat carbohydrate (sugars and starches), our bodies convert it into glucose. Some of the foods rich in carbohydrate are:

- breads, cereals and biscuits
- pulses (such as dried peas, beans and lentils)
- starchy vegetables (such as potatoes)
- rice and pasta
- fruit
- milk
- sugar
- foods with sugar added, such as cakes, sweet biscuits, confectionery, sweetened soft drinks and canned fruit.

The digestive system breaks down carbohydrate to make glucose and other sugars. The sugars are then absorbed into the bloodstream directly from the digestive tract or gut.

What happens to the glucose?

The blood carries the glucose to your body tissues (for instance, your lungs, heart, kidneys and muscles). There, the glucose passes from your blood into the tiny cells that make up body tissues, but the only way in which this can happen is with the help of the hormone insulin. On the wall of each tiny cell are special key holes or receptor sites. The insulin attaches itself to the glucose in the blood and locks itself into the receptor site in much the same way as you would use a key to open a door. This allows the glucose to pass through the cell wall into the cell where it is used for fuel.

Insulin is produced by the pancreas, a small gland that lies behind the stomach. Scattered throughout the pancreas are clusters of specialised cells, the Islets of Langerhans, which make and store insulin, and then release it into the bloodstream as needed. The pancreas, despite its small size, also produces digestive juices which help your body break down food as it passes through the gut.

After you have eaten, digested and absorbed food containing carbohydrate, the amount of glucose in your blood increases. In response to this, the pancreas releases the correct amount of insulin into your blood to carry the extra glucose into the cells. The amount of glucose in your blood then returns to its pre-meal level. At least, that's the way the system is supposed to work. If you don't have diabetes, your blood glucose level never goes too high or too low, no matter how much or how little carbohydrate you eat. The system balances itself.

What happens when diabetes develops?

When the body produces little or no insulin, or the insulin it does produce is unable to carry glucose into your body cells, you develop diabetes.

With your normal glucose regulating system out of order, your level of blood glucose keeps on increasing. When it reaches a certain level, the body attempts to tackle the problem by passing the extra glucose out of your body via your urine. This is called 'glycosuria'—literally 'glucose urine'. Not surprisingly, with it can come symptoms such as:

- passing large amounts of urine by day and night. This is called polyuria meaning 'much urine', and nocturia meaning 'night urine' as a way of getting rid of the excess sugar;
- feeling very thirsty most of the time and having a dry mouth, the result of the large urine output;
- drinking excessively (polydipsia) in response to thirst;
- excessive tiredness due to the lack of available fuel to the cells;
- losing weight because the normal fuel, glucose, is not available and the body breaks down fat stores;
- itchiness and infections resulting from bacteria feeding on the extra glucose in blood and urine;
- blurring of vision due to the effect of the high blood glucose on the fluid levels in the eye. A medical examination will then reveal a high blood glucose level, in other words, a diagnosis of diabetes.

A high blood glucose level is known as hyperglycaemia, from 'hyper', meaning excessive and 'glycaemia' for sugar in the blood.

TYPES OF DIABETES

There are 2 main types of diabetes:

- Type 1 diabetes;
- Type 2 diabetes;

Other types of diabetes include:

- gestational diabetes;
- diabetes that results from genetic abnormalities, biological or metabolic events or certain medications used to treat other conditions.

Type 1 diabetes
(until recently referred to as Insulin-Dependent Diabetes Mellitus—IDDM)

This type of diabetes results from damage or deterioration in pancreatic function that leads to a complete lack of insulin production. It is estimated that about 10–15 per cent of Britons with diabetes have this type.

Type 1 diabetes can develop at any age, but is more common in childhood, during the teens or in early adulthood. What causes it is still unknown, but it may be caused by a virus which leads to the destruction of the Islets of Langerhans within the pancreas. Whatever the cause, the pancreas stops making insulin and symptoms usually appear quickly and severely.

If not treated promptly, your blood glucose level rises. As the glucose cannot get into the cells, your body begins burning up its fat stores too quickly (ketosis) and your breath smells of acetone. You may vomit, become dehydrated and feel drowsy. Left untreated, you will eventually lapse into a coma.

The treatment is a combination of insulin injections and the healthy diet we present in this book. It is necessary to inject insulin, because if you were to take it by mouth it would be destroyed by your digestive juices long before it could be absorbed and used.

Type 2 diabetes
(until recently referred to as Non-Insulin-Dependent Diabetes Mellitus—NIDDM)

This is the major type of diabetes both in the UK and worldwide and results from an insufficiency in insulin production and/or a resistance to its action. It develops slowly and symptoms, if any, are likely to be less extreme than with Type 1 diabetes. The only sign may be a high blood glucose level (hyperglycaemia) picked up on routine testing by your doctor.

Type 2 diabetes usually develops in people over the age of forty. It accounts for between 75 – 90 per cent of all cases. There is often a family history of diabetes. A number of factors may influence the development of Type 2 diabetes, most importantly:

- family history
- age
- overweight
- stress
- alcohol abuse
- inactivity.

With this type of diabetes, the pancreas makes some insulin, but not enough. Alternatively, other factors such as excess body fat restricts the action of the insulin carrying glucose into the body's cells (often referred to as insulin resistance).

Treatment for Type 2 diabetes involves a healthy diet and exercise. For the overweight person with this type of diabetes, losing weight is the most important part of treatment. If this is not enough to control the blood glucose then oral medication or insulin may be given.

Even with well-controlled diabetes, insulin or extra oral medication may be needed during periods of illness, emotional distress or after surgery. With time, the pancreatic function of people with diabetes frequently deteriorates and despite a healthy lifestyle, medication may need to be used to help with the control of blood glucose.

Gestational diabetes

It is difficult to establish how many women develop this during pregnancy. It is caused by increased levels of some hormones that decrease the effectiveness of the insulin's action in helping glucose pass into the tissues.

Although it usually disappears on the baby's birth, some women with gestational diabetes will develop Type 2 diabetes later on in life. The diabetes should be well controlled during pregnancy and a healthy lifestyle maintained after the baby's birth. Medical follow up, at least two-yearly, may be necessary in the long term.

Impaired Glucose Tolerance

In addition, there are many people who have blood glucose levels above the normal range but not high enough to be diagnosed with diabetes. These people are described as having impaired glucose tolerance.

As with diabetes, a healthy eating pattern, regular exercise and long-term weight control is necessary for those with impaired glucose tolerance. With this about a third will improve, a third will remain glucose intolerant and a third will develop Type 2 diabetes.

HOW IS DIABETES DIAGNOSED?

Anyone showing symptoms and everyone over sixty-five years of age or with two or more risk factors should be tested for diabetes.

Risk factors include being over forty, a family history of diabetes, high risk ethnic groups (e.g. Aboriginal background, Indian and Maltese immigrants), presence of obesity, high blood pressure, high blood fat levels and history of gestational diabetes.

Diagnosis is made by simple blood test, either fasting, random or post prandial. Fasting blood glucose is checked when you have been without food or drink for ten to twelve hours. A random test is done at any time regardless of whether you have eaten or not. Post prandial is taken two hours after eating.

Blood Glucose Levels

The fasting blood glucose level for a person without diabetes is considered to be between 3.5 and 5.9 mmol/litre and a random level less than 7.8 mmol/litre, however the diagnosis criteria are stricter depending on presence of symptoms or risk factors. The following criteria are used to determine diabetes:

DIAGNOSIS MMOL/LITRE	FASTING GLUCOSE MMOL/LITRE	POST PRANDIAL MANAGEMENT	COMMENT, ONGOING
Diabetes unlikely	<5.5	<5.5	Should retest 1–5 yearly depending on risk factors
Presence of impaired glucose tolerance uncertain	5.5–6.0	5.5–6.9	Further investigation needed. May confirm impaired glucose tolerance
Impaired glucose tolerance	6.1–6.9	7.0–11	
Diabetes	> 7.0	> 11	Diabetes likely, may be confirmed with further blood test
Gestational diabetes	> 5.4	> 7.9	

There are a variety of other blood tests available where further testing is needed to confirm a diagnosis. One test is the glucose tolerance test where a fasting blood test is performed, then 75g of glucose is given orally and further blood samples tested one and two hours afterwards.

A blood test frequently used which reflects long-term blood glucose control is known as the HbA1c (glycosylated haemoglobin). This is sometimes used as a diagnostic tool but more frequently to determine control in people with diabetes. The following criteria are used to assess control:

- normal range 4.7–6.1%
- good control 6.2–8.0%
- fair control 8.1–10.0%
- poor control >10.0%

DIABETES TABLETS AND HOW THEY WORK

Diabetes tablets (oral hypoglycaemic agents) help lower your blood glucose level. They don't contain insulin, but help the body make more insulin or help you use the insulin you have more effectively.

What happens if diabetes remains uncontrolled?

If your blood glucose level remains high or fluctuates excessively over a period, this may damage the blood vessels that supply your eyes, kidneys, heart and other organs and nerves, especially in your legs and feet. Learning how to manage your diabetes and to achieve good control is the best way to avoid these complications.

MANAGING DIABETES TODAY

Essentially, good management of diabetes focuses on three major approaches:
- diet
- diet and diabetes tablets
- diet and insulin injections.

Exactly which approach is most beneficial for you will depend on what type of diabetes you have, your weight, age and your blood glucose level. Regular exercise makes an important difference to all people with diabetes and to your sense of well-being and general health.

There are two other important guidelines which will keep you fit and in good health:
- regular monitoring of your blood glucose levels helps you get to know your body and how it is coping with diabetes. It shows you the effect food, exercise and medication have on your blood glucose level (BGL), and helps you adjust them as necessary;
- regular visits to your doctor, dietitian and/or diabetes nurse—your partners in ongoing health care.

What can diet do for diabetes?

Food is important in keeping healthy, whether we have diabetes or not. However, most people don't pay enough attention to their basic nutritional needs. Diabetes highlights the importance of a well-balanced eating pattern. If you have diabetes, there are three important benefits to be had from a nutritionally sound diet:
- firstly, it helps you achieve and maintain good control of your blood glucose level;
- secondly, it helps you regulate your body weight;
- thirdly, it helps prevent or delay the onset of the long-term problems linked with diabetes.

THE GOLDEN RULES FOR DIABETES

The way to keep healthy now and in the future is to follow these golden rules:

1. Understand your diabetes and how to manage it

Ask questions. Don't be shy or worry that you seem 'stupid' or are being a bother. No matter how 'silly' your question, ask it. And keep on asking until you are entirely satisfied that you understand your diabetes and know what to do to manage it. If, like so many people, you tend to go blank when seeing the dietitian, doctor or diabetes educator, sit down before your visit and write out all your questions and concerns. Take your list with you and go through it item by item.

These people are often busy and, if you need extra time, make an appointment for a less busy time. Alternatively, ask for a double appointment. Make sure you understand exactly what the prescribed treatment is supposed to do, and exactly how to follow it. You can also take a parent, friend or partner to help you remember what was said.

2. Keep your blood glucose level under control

The best way of doing this is to eat sensibly, exercise regularly and take your medication correctly. Check your blood glucose levels regularly and have your doctor or diabetes educator do this at regular intervals.

3. If you are overweight, make losing weight a goal

If you are a healthy weight, stay that way. There is no magic to losing weight. Basically, you need to make sure that you choose a low-fat diet and eat fewer kilojoules (calories) than your body burns up. You probably know whether you are eating too much, but if you are unsure of how to cut down on kilojoules (calories) without losing out on good nutrition, look at the meal plans in this book.

Once you are a healthy weight, keep a careful watch on what you eat; it's all a matter of balance. You need to eat just enough to fuel your body through its normal daily routine. Concentrate on those things that provide your body with enough nutrients to keep it functioning perfectly and continue to choose low-fat meals. Remember, you can do this and still enjoy varied and tasty meals.

4. Be as physically active as possible

Keep in mind your age, general health and your ability to exercise. This is not a call to becoming a super-athlete; simply by taking a brisk walk round the block twice a day you can keep fit. You may prefer to swim a few laps, play bowls or tennis, ride your bicycle or walk to the local shops instead of driving. But whatever exercise you choose, and whatever level of physical activity you find most comfortable, make it a regular part of your life. The benefits are immense.

UNDERSTANDING THE PRINCIPLES OF GOOD NUTRITION

Food is an important part of life—it is a necessity and it should be a pleasure. Diabetes need not change either of these aspects.

What we eat is a very individual matter. It's one of those areas where personal choice is allowed a wide expression. How you feel at any particular moment, your tastes, your cultural background and lifestyle, all have an effect on your food choices.

The enjoyment we get from food should be matched by its value as a source of nourishment. It's the sort of thing we all are becoming more aware of, but may well ignore. However, when you develop diabetes, you have the opportunity to reappraise what you eat and improve your eating habits with immediate and significant benefits.

Foods provide a range of different textures, flavours, colours and nutritional value, and eating a variety will ensure the best combination for good health. The nutrients in food include protein, fat, carbohydrate, vitamins, minerals, fibre and water, all of which are essential for continued good health. We now know that there are other components in foods that may have a health protection function, such as phytochemicals (plant chemicals). These components in some foods seem to have 'antioxidant' properties. It may be of help to know what these different food components do, and why they are vital.

Protein

- An important part of all body tissues, enzymes, hormones and the immune system.
- You need protein for body growth and repair.
- It has only a small role as a body fuel.
- The richest sources are meat, poultry, fish, seafood, dairy products, eggs, pulses, nuts, seeds and tofu. You don't have to eat huge quantities of protein to meet your body needs.

Fat

- Provides fuel to keep the body working.
- Plays an important part in insulating and protecting the body's organs and other tissues.
- Transports other nutrients (especially vitamins A, D, E and K) into and around the body.
- You need small amounts to provide essential fatty acids which the body cannot make. These perform inportant tasks. Major sources of fat include butter, margarine and other spreads, oils, all meats and poultry, cheese, full-cream milk and yoghurt and nuts.
- Fried and takeaway foods, dips, potato crisps, snack foods, cream, ice-cream, many dressings and sauces, most cakes, biscuits, pastries and chocolate all contain large amounts of fats and should be limited.
- There are different types of fats in foods and these become significant when considering blood fat levels and heart disease—see page 42.

Carbohydrate

- The most important fuel source for all body tissues, especially the brain.
- Plays an important part in many body functions.
- Comes in two main forms—sugars and starches. Sugars are found naturally in fruit, milk and honey, and are added as sweeteners to many foods such as confectionery, cakes, soft drinks and jams. You find starches in breads, cereals, grains, vegetables and pulses.

Vitamins

- Help the body produce fuel from carbohydrate, fat and protein.
- Work in combination with protein in growth and repair of body tissues.
- Play an essential part in body functions.
- There are two types of vitamins: water-soluble vitamins, that is, all B vitamins and Vitamin C, which are found widely in foods including fruits, vegetables, cereals, milk and meat; and fat-soluble vitamins—A, D, E and K—which are found in animal fats such as butter, other dairy products, meat, fish, vegetable oils and margarines, wholegrain products, nuts and seeds.

Minerals

- Form a major part of bones, teeth and body fluids such as blood.
- Play an essential part in body functions such as heart beat, muscle contraction, and in the nervous system and fluid balance.
- Occur widely in foods such as meat and fish, milk and cheese, fruits, vegetables and cereals.

Fibre

- Used to be called roughage and is the part of plant foods which is not broken down by the digestive juices.
- It has several functions, including keeping the digestive tract in good shape. In other words, it keeps our bowels functioning regularly and easily.
- Also helps fill the stomach, satisfies our appetite and helps to limit over-eating.
- Delays the onset of hunger by slowing both digestion and the rate at which our body absorbs nutrients. In particular, from the point of view of a person with diabetes, it slows the rate of absorption of carbohydrate from the gut, thereby helping to control the blood glucose level.
- Fibre is invaluable in your diet. Eat lots of it. Good sources of fibre include wholegrain breads and cereals, fruits, vegetables and pulses.

Water

- An essential part of every body function. About two-thirds of the body is water.
- We lose between one and three litres of water every day through the lungs and in urine, faeces and sweat. The body can survive only for a few days without replacing this loss.
- Water is the best drink for health. Don't wait until you're thirsty. Drink at least six to eight cups of fluid a day, and you will feel the benefit.

Phytochemicals (Antioxidants)

- Studies show that populations that eat a diet high in plant foods have a lower incidence of certain diseases including many cancers, cardiovascular disorders and diabetes.
- Each plant food contains hundreds of biologically active compounds. Currently 12 000 phytochemicals have been identified in foods.
- Phytochemicals are known to have antioxidant properties ie. protect us from potentially harmful compounds known as 'free radicals'. It is thought that 'free radicals' may damage cells, leading to degenerative diseases such as cancer, heart disease and some eye disorders.
- Rich sources of antioxidants include fruits and vegetables. Pulses, including soybeans, tea, red and white wine, nuts and olive oil are also useful sources.

Food as a fuel source

Food is the energy source or fuel that keeps our bodies working. The energy supplied by any food is measured in kilojoules (or calories). Energy comes from three particular nutrients in our food: carbohydrate, fat and protein.

Alcohol provides concentrated energy, but it isn't usually considered a nutrient and isn't essential.

The general recommendation is to encourage plenty of variety in food choice. A small amount of a wide range of foods may well offer more health protection than eating larger amounts of a limited range of foods.

GUIDELINES FOR CHOOSING FOOD

Dietary recommendations for people with diabetes are very similar to those aimed at the general population for the promotion of good health. In 1999, a group of European nutrition experts in the field of diabetes published updated dietary guidelines. This section is based mainly on these recommendations and explains why they are important to you.

- Maintain a healthy weight. If overweight, aim to lose weight, or if this is difficult, avoid further weight gain.
- Take part in regular, moderate physical activity most days of the week.
- Base meals around starchy high fibre foods.
- Eat five or more servings of fruit and vegetables every day.
- Eat less fat, especially saturated and trans fats. Substitute these fats with mainly monounsaturated fat and some polyunsaturated fat.
- Moderate intakes of sugar can be included as part of a healthy diet.
- Limit salt intake to under 6g/day.
- If you drink alcohol, keep within sensible limits.

Maintain a healthy body weight

Being overweight makes diabetes more difficult to control. The extra body fat alters the cell receptor sites, as described on pages 5–6, so that they are unable to accept the combination of insulin and glucose. As a result, blood glucose levels remain too high.

Fortunately, once you lose excess weight, the receptor sites are reactivated, allowing insulin to be taken up effectively so that your blood glucose level can be better controlled. Even modest weight loss can help to improve your blood glucose levels.

If you are overweight, losing weight is the key to good diabetes control, and should be a priority. It will also benefit your overall health. Check the following chart to see whether you need to maintain or lose weight.

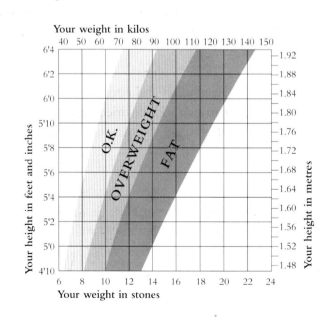

Whether you need to maintain or lose weight, the guidelines given in this book will help you achieve your goal. In order to lose weight you will have to reduce your total energy (calorie) intake, and increase energy output, by being more physically active.

By limiting your fat and sugar intake, and having more starchy, high-fibre foods and fruit and vegetables, you should be able to control your weight and still eat enough to satisfy your appetite.

While you are losing weight, it is important to maintain your health by eating regular meals that supply all your nutritional needs. Avoid crash diets and quick solutions—they offer no long-term benefits. Developing a healthy eating pattern over a long period of time will help you to achieve and maintain a lower weight.

Take part in regular physical activity

Being physically active is one good way to improve everyone's health. It is particularly important when you have diabetes, because being active is likely to:

- improve blood glucose control;
- improve the balance of blood fats (lipids);
- help with weight loss and weight maintenance.

Guidelines for being more physically active:

- Try to be more active on at least 5 days of the week, and work towards 30 minutes of moderate physical activity, such as walking ('moderate' means moving about enough to make you feel warm and slightly out of breath);
- Build up gradually and aim for 15-30 minutes at a time, although every bit of activity helps;
- Choose an activity you enjoy such as walking, gardening, swimming, dancing, heavy DIY;
- If in doubt about how much activity is right for you, speak to your doctor first.

Base meals around starchy, high fibre foods

These foods offer a number of benefits and should make up the bulk of your diet (approximately half your daily energy). They contain energy in the form of carbohydrate, fibre, vitamins and minerals and, if you eat them regularly, will help control your diabetes. They can also help with weight management. Include some of the following with each meal:

- **Bread, cereals and potatoes:** include all types of bread, breakfast cereals, rice, oats, pasta (such as spaghetti and noodles), maize, millet and cornmeal.
- **Pulses and beans (also called legumes):** include dried beans (such as red kidney, borlotti, black-eyed, haricot, cannellini, baked beans and soy beans), peas (such as split peas and chick peas) and lentils.

Carbohydrate and diabetes

Knowing about carbohydrate is important for you if you have diabetes. After all, carbohydrate breaks down into glucose, and balancing your blood glucose level is a vital part of your management. It is important to include at least three or four serves of high-carbohydrate, high-fibre food in every meal. If you are young and/or active, your carbohydrate requirements will be much higher. You may find that you need more carbohydrate at meals and/or high-carbohydrate snacks to ensure you have enough carbohydrate in your body all through the day.

The following information on the Glycaemic Index will show you that two foods with the same amount of carbohydrate may have quite different effects on your blood glucose levels and therefore food does not need to be accurately measured or weighed. We use average servings as a basis for carbohydrate intake. Experience has shown that as long you are consistent this can give you good control and make life easier.

It is useful for you to understand that foods high in added sugars are often low in nutrients and may be high in fat, whereas the carbohydrate-rich foods which are high in natural sugars and starches—such as breads, cereals, some vegetables, pulses and fruit—provide many essential nutrients and fibre, as well as energy. They should form the basis of your eating plan.

The Glycaemic Index

Serves of different carbohydrate foods have different effects on the blood glucose levels, even when they provide the same amount of carbohydrate, with some causing a quicker and higher rise in blood glucose levels than others. This is because foods are digested and/or absorbed at different rates.

Foods are rated (1–100) according to the effect they have on blood glucose levels. This is known as the Glycaemic Index (GI). Foods that are digested and absorbed slowly cause a small rise in blood glucose levels and have a low GI number. Foods that cause a greater rise have a higher GI number. The best foods for control of diabetes are those which have a low GI number, providing that they are also low in fat.

Many factors affect the Glycaemic Index such as the amount of processing, preparation and cooking, the type of sugar or starch, the amount and type of fibre and the amount of fat.

So what effect do these factors have?

- **Processing:** the more a food is processed the easier it is for the body to break down the food and absorb the carbohydrate and therefore the quicker the rise in blood glucose level. For instance, a smooth wholemeal bread has a higher GI than a heavy wholegrain bread.
- **Preparation and cooking:** the more a food is chopped up and cooked the easier it is for the body to digest and absorb the carbohydrate. For instance, stewed apple is broken down more easily than raw apple.
- **Sugar:** there are different types of sugar in our foods and each is absorbed at different rates. Glucose is absorbed very quickly and has a very high GI. Fructose or fruit sugar is absorbed slowly and has a low GI. Sucrose or cane sugar, the sugar we commonly use in the kitchen, is a mixture of glucose and fructose and has a medium GI.
- **Starch:** starch is made up of glucose joined together in chains. These chains come in different forms. Some starches are broken down and absorbed more quickly than others. For instance, the starch in short grain rice is absorbed more quickly than the starch in most pastas.
- **Fibre:** fibre helps to slow down the digestion and absorption of starches. Not only is the amount of fibre in a food relevant but also the type of fibre. For instance, the fibre in oats and bran slows absorption.

- **Fat:** foods high in fats often have a low GI. This is because fat slows digestion. However, a high fat intake is not recommended for people with diabetes.

Include foods of low GI regularly in your diet to help control of blood glucose levels. It is recommended that at least one food of low GI (as listed below) be included at each meal. For those who eat between meals, it is best to choose low GI snacks.

Most foods with a high GI may also be eaten regularly as they provide important nutrients and variety to our food intake. Combining foods of low GI with those of high GI helps to even out swings in blood glucose levels and leads to better control. Individual responses to foods can vary—speak to your dietitian if you are concerned.

The foods that offer the most benefit to people with diabetes in terms of GI include:
- pulses/legumes (all varieties);
- oats; oat, barley, wheat and rice bran cereals;
- wholemeal/granary breads and wholegrain rye bread;
- barley, buckwheat, bulgar;
- all wheat-based pastas including spaghetti and noodles;
- fruits such as apples, cherries, grapes, grapefruit, oranges, peaches, pears, plums and firm bananas;
- some vegetables such as sweet potatoes, yam and sweetcorn;
- some long grain rice such as basmati;
- low fat milk and yoghurt.

The food value lists on pages 208–214 show the Glycaemic Index of many foods, along with the carbohydrate, fat and energy levels and may be used as a guide to food choice.

By using the Glycaemic Index rating carbohydrate-rich foods can be classified as high GI (index number of 70 or more), medium GI (index number between 55–70) or low GI (index number of 55 or less). This information is current, but research continues and there may be further changes.

Fibre

As mentioned earlier, fibre is important in helping to control your blood glucose level and regulating bowel function. Some fibres (known as 'soluble') may also help lower blood cholesterol. To maximise your fibre intake:
- choose wholegrain/wholemeal or oat-based breakfast cereals;
- choose wholegrain/wholemeal, rye or high fibre breads;
- replace white rice and pastas with brown rice and wholewheat pastas—you'll be delighted with how tasty they are;
- use more pulses in your cooking. Add them to soups, casseroles, salads, savoury dishes and dips;
- include plenty of vegetables every day (including the starchy ones). Use them in salads, soups, meat dishes and so on;
- include at least two to three pieces of fruit in your daily eating plan. Preferably eat them fresh rather than cooked, and don't drink more than one small glass of fruit juice per day, as this is low in fibre;
- leave vegetables and fruit unpeeled where possible, for maximum fibre.

Eat five or more servings of fruit and vegetables every day

Include a variety of fresh, frozen, canned fruit (in fruit juice), vegetables and dried fruit. A glass of fruit juice can also contribute. These foods are naturally rich in antioxidants (especially vitamin C, beta-carotene (which can be converted to vitamin A in the body) and vitamin E). They are also a good source of fibre and folate (a B vitamin).

Eat less fat

Fat is a taste-enhancer and adds texture to many foods. It also provides fat-soluble vitamins and essential fatty acids. Unfortunately, we have become used to eating too much of it. Not only do we use it knowingly by frying foods or by ladling on the cream; we also eat a great deal of fat unknowingly in processed foods. It is sobering to realise that a 30g packet of potato crisps contains almost 40 per cent fat and 165 kcal and that a plain biscuit may have as much as 20 per cent fat and 70 kcal.

Fat is the most concentrated form of energy we eat, providing more than twice the amount of calories per gram than both carbohydrate and protein. There is a danger that a diet high in fats will lead to excessive weight gain.

Heart and circulation problems are often associated with a diet high in saturated and trans fats. Reduce your intake of these fats and this may reduce your chances of developing such problems. Small amounts of oils and foods such as lean meats, low fat dairy foods and wholegrain cereal products will provide adequate amounts of fats for health. Monounsaturated fats (eg. olive oil) and small amounts of polyunsaturated fats (eg. sunflower oil) are good substitutes for saturated fat (see p. 42 for more details).

Excessive fat stores in the body and large amounts of fat in the diet can increase insulin resistance by inhibiting insulin activity. This will cause an increase in your blood glucose levels. Reducing dietary fat, particularly saturated and trans fats, is important for most people with diabetes. This is especially important where overweight is a problem.

Where a person with diabetes is underweight, weight gain can be beneficial for good health. An increase in fat intake and in particular unsaturated fats, may be recommended. This may be particularly important in elderly people where limited appetite can lead to under nutrition.

Just as you don't have to give up the sweetness in your foods, you don't have to give up fats altogether. It is important, however, that you limit your intake. Cutting back begins in the kitchen, and continues at the table.

Hints to help you use less fat

- Select small servings of lean meats or poultry; trim away visible fat and remove skin; try to include two to three servings of fish (especially oil-rich fish) per week.
- Use low-fat dairy products—milks, cheeses, yoghurts, ice-creams—in preference to the full fat varieties.
- Spread margarine or butter very lightly on bread or switch to a reduced- or low-fat spread.
- If desired, a cheese spread, a reduced-fat dip, pickles, chutney or reduced-fat mayonnaise may be used sparingly to replace margarine or butter.
- Use salad dressings sparingly or use oil-free varieties instead. Also good to add zest to your salads is lemon juice or balsamic vinegar with herbs. Turn to the 'sauces and dressings' section (page 161) for ideas.
- Use a pure vegetable oil (such as olive or sunflower) in cooking. If possible, don't use any added fat at all.
- When you do use fat or oil, use less than the recipe suggests or use a cooking spray or brush to spread a thin layer of fat onto the pan.
- Onions, garlic, spices or herbs can be sautéd in water or stock.
- For soups and casseroles, drop meat into boiling water to seal it rather that browning it in fat or oil. When cooked cool quickly, refrigerate and skim fat off the top when it hardens.
- Grill or bake meat on a rack to allow fat to drain away.
- Roast or bake vegetables in stock or in foil, with herbs and garlic or try dry baking them in the oven in their own skins.
- Stir-fry vegetables in a little oil, or stock.
- Experiment with fresh or dried herbs, spices, onion, tomato or lemon juice to add flavour to food rather than butter or oil.
- Avoid adding oil or fat to vegetables during or after preparation. For instance, mash potatoes or other vegetables with low-fat milk or stock.
- Use low-fat custard sauce, yoghurt, or low-fat ice-cream instead of cream on desserts.
- Save cream for special occasions and then use it in small amounts.
- Read food labels carefully; learn to choose lower-fat products. In the section 'making sense of food labels', on page 24, we tell you how best to choose low-fat foods when shopping.

Our recipes reflect our recommendations; we use fat where necessary, but sparingly. The recipes will convince you that you can eat wonderful, nutritious food and still cut down on fat.

Protein foods

Protein foods often contain fat, so be aware of this when you make choices. Consider the following:

- **Meat, poultry and fish:** protein is important to a healthy eating plan and you should include some every day. Most people eat far too much. You only need one or two small servings of protein foods daily. By a small serving, we mean about 75–85g (3oz) of cooked meat or fish. To give you some idea of what this means, it's equivalent to 2 small slices of cooked meat.

  If in doubt at first, weigh your meats or fish, or ask your butcher or fishmonger to weigh them for you. When choosing protein foods, select those which are lower in fat, such as: lean beef, pork or lamb; fish and seafood; chicken or turkey without skin; lean game meat such as pheasant. To be classified as lean, meat should have minimal visible fat marbled through it, and you should trim off any fat around the meat before you cook it.

- **Eggs:** eggs are a good source of protein. They are low in fat, although the yolk is rich in cholesterol. As part of a healthy diet you can eat three or four eggs a week. Two eggs make a good serving size.

- **Pulses:** pulses are excellent as a source of protein and have the added advantage of being low in fat. They make an ideal alternative or addition to meat dishes. They are rich in carbohydrate and fibre, so include them often. About 100g (4oz) of cooked (or canned) pulses is a good serving size.

- **Nuts and seeds:** nuts and seeds—and products made from them, such as peanut butter and tahini—are a valuable source of protein, but are high in fat, so eat them in small amounts.

- **Tofu (soybean curd):** the use of tofu is growing in popularity with the introduction of Asian style recipes and with the increasing recognition of the health benefits of soy products. It is low in fat and rich in protein and B-vitamins. It is bland to taste but readily absorbs the flavour of other foods during cooking. The consistency of tofu can vary and is described as being firm, soft or silken: firm tofu is dense and can be cubed and added to stir-fries and soups; soft tofu tends to fall apart more easily and is good for blending; silken tofu is soft and creamy and can be used to replace cream or sour cream in savoury recipes and in dips.

- **Milk and milk products:** whole milk and dairy products can be high in fat, but there are many low-fat products available such as skimmed or semi-skimmed milks; low-fat yoghurts, natural or artificially sweetened; reduced-fat cheeses; reduced-fat ice-creams.

Milk and yoghurt contain the carbohydrate lactose (milk sugar). The use of small amounts of milk such as that taken in tea or coffee need not be considered as a carbohydrate source, but a glass of milk or a carton of yoghurt makes a good alternative to other carbohydrate foods.

A SPECIAL NOTE ON MILK AND DAIRY FOODS

Dairy products are important sources of protein and calcium. Women, particularly, should be aware of the value of dairy products in helping protect them from osteoporosis (loss of calcium from bones, making them brittle). Calcium, of course, plays a vital part in good bone health.

To meet calcium needs, adults should aim to eat 2–3 servings of dairy foods every day. Children, adolescents, and women who are pregnant, breast-feeding or post-menopausal have higher requirements. The following serving sizes each contain about the same quantity of calcium:
  • 1 third pint (200ml) of milk • 1 carton of yoghurt • 40g piece of cheese

Moderate intakes of sugar can be included

If liked, moderate intakes of sugar can be included as part of your healthy diet, whether you have Type 1 or Type 2 diabetes. As for the general population, it's a good idea to limit the amount of added sugar, as sugar is relatively high in calories but low in other nutrients. This means that sugary foods can add to your energy intake without providing useful nourishment. You will find sugar in many forms, some obvious, some less so, in many of the foods you buy such as cereals, biscuits, canned fruit, soft drinks, confectionery and chocolate.

In practice, the best way to use sugar rich foods is to use less of them, such as spreading just a small amount of jam on wholegrain toast or adding a little sugar to a wholemeal cake recipe.

Hints to help you cut down on sugar
  • Always check product labels. Read the section 'making sense of food labels' (page 24).
  • Avoid sugar in tea, coffee or other beverages.
  • Buy fruit canned in water or natural juice instead of fruit canned in syrups.
  • Water is the best thirst quencher. Alternatively choose 'diet' (low-calorie) soft drinks, flavoured mineral waters and cordials instead of the regular varieties.
  • If you want flavoured jellies, choose the 'diet' (low-calorie) varieties.
  • If you like jam, marmalade or honey on your toast or bread, have some, but limit it to a scrape.
  • In your cooking, look for recipes with only small amounts of sugar or honey. Our recipes will give you a guide to just how little sugar or sweetness you need to make food delicious. Remember, too, that fruit (particularly dried) is a good source of sweetness. In many of our recipes you will see that we use fruit and fruit juices in recipes which traditionally are made with sugar.
  • Low-fat fruit yoghurts are often surprisingly high in sugar. Choose 'diet' or low calorie varieties and limit any sweetened ones to mealtimes. Try making your own by combining low-fat natural yoghurt and your choice of fresh or stewed fruits.
  • There are several artificial sweeteners on the market. These may be used to replace sugar.

Limit salt intake

We all eat too much salt in the UK, so recommendations to limit salt intake to about 6g/day (approximately 1 teaspoon) applies to people with diabetes too. If you have high blood pressure, it may be advisable to cut down on salt even further than this. See pages 41–42 for hints on how to reduce dietary salt.

Limit the amount of alcohol you drink

Alcoholic drinks are high in calories and can contribute to weight gain. Having diabetes does not mean that you cannot drink alcohol at all. If you drink alcohol, it simply means drink it in moderation and with good sense.

Recent research has indicated that various components of alcoholic beverages, including antioxidants, may offer health protection.

A moderate intake is considered to be up to 21 units spread throughout the week for women and up to 28 units spread throughout the week for men. One unit of alcohol is equivalent to:

- a single measure of spirits such as whisky, brandy, gin, vodka
- a small glass of sherry, vermouth, port
- 120ml (small glass) of wine
- half a pint of ordinary beer or lager.

Intakes greater than these can have adverse effects on health.

Remember that all alcoholic drinks are high in calories. Sweet varieties of wines, sherries, vermouth, port and all liquers contain sugar and are higher in calories than drier varieties.

Don't be lulled into a false sense of security by drinking 'diet' beers. Although lower in carbohydrate, these contain as much alcohol and have similar calorie contents as regular beers. They should be treated as if they were ordinary alcoholic drinks when it comes to quantity. It is best to drink low alcohol (less than three per cent alcohol) beers rather than regular beers as these are lower in calories. Watch out for strong beers and lagers – they have a higher alcohol content.

There are many new types of beers presently being introduced. If you are uncertain about their content, check with your dietitian before including them in your diet. Rather than a regular mixer, a low-calorie slimline soft drink, soda water or plain mineral water mixed with spirits will help lower calorie and sugar intake. Soda water mixed with wine makes a longer drink. It is always a good idea to drink a glass of water along with an alcoholic drink.

If you are taking hypoglycaemic (diabetes) tablets or insulin, and you drink alcohol without having carbohydrate, the alcohol may react with your medication and your blood glucose levels may drop too low. This may lead to hypoglycaemia (low blood sugars). Don't drink alcohol on an empty stomach. Always eat some starchy food when you drink, for example, wine with a meal. Fruit juice and milk contain carbohydrate and are useful mixers. Be aware that regular soft drinks contain large amounts of sugar and have a higher glycaemic index than either fruit juice or milk. On page 39 we tell you more about hypoglycaemia, how to prevent and treat it. You will find more information on alcohol on page 214.

REMEMBER, IN YOUR QUEST FOR BETTER HEALTH:

- eat regular meals each day;
- include plenty of wholegrain bread, cereals, pasta and pulses every day;
- aim for 5 or more servings of fruit and vegetables daily;
- limit fats, concentrated sugars and alcohol;
- aim to lose weight if you are overweight; if you are a healthy weight, aim to keep it that way;
- eating should be a pleasure; make sure your meals have plenty of flavour and texture.

ON THE SHELVES

MAKING SENSE OF FOOD LABELS

Many commercial foods which you buy at the supermarket contain a lot of fat and/or sugar and may be low in fibre. But how do you know which ones they are? Reading labels provides valuable information about a product but is not always as straightforward as it looks. You need to know how to interpret the information so you can make wise choices. There are two parts to the nutrition panel that help you: the ingredient list and the nutrition information.

Ingredient lists

There are food labelling laws in the UK which state that all ingredients in a product must appear on the label, and in order of decreasing quantity. This means the ingredient used in the greatest amount is listed first, and that used in the smallest amount is listed last.

For example, let us look at a product label including the following ingredients: wheat flour, oats, animal fat, malt extract, sultanas, flavouring, salt. There is more wheat flour in this product than anything else, and less salt.

Fat, sugar, salt and fibre may be listed under a variety of differing names i.e. they may be difficult to always recognise. This can add confusion when assessing a food product as like ingredients can be spread through the label. The following names may appear on labels:

Fat
Animal fat, butter fat, cocoa fat, coconut cream, coconut oil, corn oil, hydrogenated vegetable oil, lard, lecithin, vegetable fat, vegetable oil, sunflower oil, olive oil, rapeseed oil, palm oil, soya oil.

Sugar
Brown sugar, concentrated fruit juice, corn syrup, dextrose, fructose, glucose, glucose syrup, golden syrup, apple concentrate, grape concentrate, honey, invert sugar, lactose, malt, malt extract, maltose, mannitol, modified maize starch, molasses, sorbitol, sucrose, treacle.

Salt
Celery salt, cooking salt, herb salt, lemon salt, monosodium glutamate (MSG) or flavour enhancer 621, onion salt, rock salt, sea salt, sodium bicarbonate, sodium chloride, sodium nitrate, soy sauce, table salt, vegetable salt.

Fibre
Wheat bran, oat bran, psyllium husks, rice bran, rolled oats, wheatgerm, wholegrain, wholemeal, wholewheat.

A nutrient that appears in the first two or three listed ingredients often helps to determine the suitability of a product for use in a given diet as the product may contain large amounts of the ingredient. However, this can also be misleading as the level of the second or third ingredient may only be there in relatively small amounts when compared with the quantity of the primary ingredient. It is therefore important to look for a nutrition information panel.

Nutrition information

Although still voluntary in the UK, many products include a chart showing nutrient composition. This information is of greater value than the ingredient list as it is more accurate and allows you to make product comparisons more easily. When included, nutrition information must be expressed in a particular way; either (a) Energy (kJ/kcal); Protein; Carbohydrate and Fat, or (b) Energy (kJ/kcal); Protein, Carbohydrate; Sugars, Fat, Saturates, Fibre and Sodium. Vitamin and mineral content are usually only declared when a claim is being made. Amounts are given 'per recommended serving' and 'per 100g' or 'per 100ml'. The 'per 100g' is the most useful for comparing foods which are of similar type. Note that grams 'per 100g' is the same as percentage. For instance 3g fat per 100g of product means that the product is three per cent fat.

Example label

Baked beans in tomato sauce (vegetarian) ingredients: beans (49%), tomatoes (27%), water, sugar, salt, modified cornflour, spirit vinegar, spice extracts, herb extract.

NUTRITION INFORMATION (BAKED BEANS)		
TYPICAL VALUES	AMOUNT PER 100g	AMOUNT PER CAN
Energy	312 kJ / 75 kcal	624 kJ / 150 kcal
Protein	4.7g	9.4g
Carbohydrate	13.6g	27.3g
(of which sugars)	(6.0g)	(12.0g)
Fat	0.2g	0.4g
(of which saturates)	(trace)	(0.1g)
Fibre	3.7g	7.4g
Sodium	0.5g	1.0g
Per Can	150 Calories	0.4g Fat

In this product, sugar appears fairly high on the list of ingredients, but on checking the nutrition information you can see that the amount of sugar per serve is quite low. Baked beans have a low GI, are also high in fibre and low in fat, making them an ideal food for people with diabetes.

Nutrition claims

The UK Government issues guidelines for manufacturers to follow when making a nutrition claim (eg. 'low fat'). The latest ones were issued in 1999, and some of the more common definitions are highlighted for you below. The best way to be confident about what is in a product, however, is to check the label yourself. If you are uncertain whether a particular product is suitable, ask your dietitian for advice.

'X% fat free' (e.g. '85% fat free')

These sort of claims can be misleading, as effectively a product which claims to be '85% fat free' still contains 15% fat! Under the latest guidelines, manufacturers can no longer make this sort of claim.

'Low fat'

To make this claim, a food product must contain no more than 3g fat per 100g/100ml. These guidelines do not apply to spreading fats, as there are specific regulations relating to these products.

'Low saturates'

Foods with this claim should contain 1.5g or less saturated fat per 100g/100ml.

'Fat free'

These claims should only be made where foods contain no more than 0.15g fat per 100g/100ml.

Cholesterol claims

'Cholesterol free', 'low cholesterol' etc. are now being phased out in line with the latest guidelines, as these are thought to mislead consumers. Cholesterol content of foods per se has little impact on blood cholesterol. It is saturated and trans fat which has the biggest dietary impact (see p.42 for more details).

'Diabetic' foods

These products are targeted at people with diabetes. Some diabetic (carbohydrate modified) chocolate, ice-cream and biscuits are high in fat. Other products include jams, chutneys, pickles and sauces which are low in fat. Generally, you will find that these specialised products are more expensive and do not taste as good as the regular variety. It is often best to use the regular products more sparingly.

SWEETENERS

As we've already mentioned, sugar does not have to be cut out of your diet completely: people with diabetes can eat sugar and still achieve good blood glucose control. Overall dietary balance is the key, and ensuring that you eat regularly.

When choosing lower sugar foods and sugar-free varieties, you are likely to eat some sweeteners, so here we offer you a guide to those on the market, and which ones are more useful when you have diabetes.

There are two types: non-intensive and intensive sweeteners.

Non-intensive sweeteners:

These include fructose and polyols (e.g. sorbitol, maltitol, mannitol, isomalt, xylitol). These type of sweeteners are not recommended for people with diabetes, as they contain calories and carbohydrate so can cause blood glucose levels to rise (like ordinary sugar). They also have a laxative effect. Non-intensive sweeteners are often found in 'diabetic' foods, sugar-free gum and sweets.

Intensive sweeteners:

These are known as artificial sweeteners and are both carbohydrate and calorie free. They include: aspartame (Nutrasweet), saccharin, acesulfame K and cyclamates. They are widely available as tablet, liquid and sprinkle sweeteners for use in drinks, on cereals and in puddings. They are also used in many manufactured foods such as low calorie yogurts; sugar free jelly, etc. As they contain no carbohydrate, they have no effect on blood glucose levels.

Examples:

Aspartame: brand names include Canderel and Hermesetas Gold.

Saccharin: brand names include Sweetex (tablets) and Original Hermesetas.

Acesulfame K: usually used in combination with other sweeteners in foods.

Cyclamate: only recently been re-introduced to the UK.

Artificial sweeteners: safety concerns?

Sweeteners are essentially food additives and as such, have to undergo safety assessments by scientific committees before an Acceptable Daily Intake (ADI) is specified. Manufacturers are also given guidance on maximum permitted levels of sweetener that can be used in specific foods. For adults, it is unlikely that they will consume quantities in excess of the ADI, but children, because of their smaller size, are more at risk.

For children: try to encourage water, milk or diluted fruit juice as drinks, in place of fizzy 'diet' drinks or low calorie squashes.

Tips and traps when using sweeteners

- Sweeteners are much sweeter than sugar, so you only need to use small amounts.
- Some people's taste buds are sensitive to these products and describe a lingering or metallic after-taste. Experiment with different types until you find one that is acceptable.
- Intensive sweeteners are not recommended for baking as they do not provide the bulk required. Try reducing the added sugar in baking recipes instead.
- Intensive sweeteners are not recommended for use in cooking when the recipe requires heating to a high temperature over a long period of time as they develop a bitter taste on heating.

PLANNING YOUR MEALS

We've given you the guidelines, now comes the application. What you choose and the quantity you eat will depend on your energy requirements and your weight, as well as on that very important factor, your preferences.

YOUR ENERGY NEEDS

The following chart shows approximate energy needs for people of different age, sex and healthy weight. If you are active your needs may be greater; if you are physically inactive your needs may be less. If you need further information or guidance discuss this with your dietitian.

ESTIMATED AVERAGE REQUIREMENTS (EAR) FOR ENERGY

AGE	EAR MJ/d (kcal/d)	
	MALES	FEMALES
11–14 years	9.27 (2,220)	7.92 (1,845)
15–18 years	11.51 (2,755)	8.83 (2,110)
19–50 years	10.60 (2,550)	8.10 (1,940)
51–59 years	10.60 (2,550)	8.00 (1,900)
60–64 years	9.93 (2,380)	7.99 (1,900)
65–74 years	9.71 (2,330)	7.96 (1,900)
75+ years	8.77 (2,100)	7.61 (1,810)
Pregnancy		+0.80 (200)
(last 3 months of pregnancy)		

YOUR CARBOHYDRATE, FAT AND PROTEIN NEEDS

The above table gives you an indication of your energy needs. As explained earlier, the nutrients which provide dietary energy are carbohydrate, fat and, to a lesser extent, protein (and alcohol). In terms of dietary balance, recommendations for the population are given for these as part of your total average energy intake, i.e.

Total fat: 30–35%
Carbohydrate: 50%
Protein: approx. 15%

So the bulk of your energy should be provided by carbohydrate, with roughly a third from fat and the rest from protein. In the UK, we tend to consume more of our calories from fat at the expense of carbohydrate.

In terms of fat, not only is total fat important, but also the quality or type of fat eaten. As a guide, no more than one third of your total daily fat intake should be from saturates, another third from polyunsaturates and the rest from monounsaturates. This equates to approximately 70g fat/day as a healthy intake for women, and 95g fat/day for men.

Currently, our intake of trans fats is around 2% of dietary energy, so we should be looking to keep this static or reduce our intake of these fats (see p. 42 for more detail).

Of course these are population average figures which should only be used as a guide. Individuals vary in terms of their energy and nutrient needs, so it would be impossible (and inappropriate) to include meal plans to suit everyone. Pages 32–35 offer some ideas and suggestions that you might like to try.

MORE ABOUT CARBOHYDRATE

For many years people with diabetes were advised to measure their carbohydrate foods accurately. Different serving sizes were used but the most common were the '10g portion' or the '15g exchange'. We now know that the serving size is less important than a meal pattern which is low in fat, moderately high in carbohydrate and fibre and with a regular intake of low Glycaemic Index foods.

It is important to eat carbohydrate foods regularly. For those on insulin injections or tablets for diabetes, it is easier to control your diabetes if you are fairly consistent in the amount and type of foods you eat from day to day but also remember variety makes meals more enjoyable.

Include at least one food of low GI per meal. Older, inactive people should eat at least three or four servings of high-carbohydrate, high-fibre foods at each of their three daily meals (45–60g of carbohydrate per meal). Younger and/or more active people may need to eat more carbohydrate portions at each meal (at least 75g of carbohydrate per meal). Remember that the high-carbohydrate, high-fibre foods include bread, cereals, pasta and pulses.

We have detailed the carbohydrate content of each recipe in this book so you know how much carbohydrate you are eating at each meal. For instance, one serve of Bombay burgers (see recipe, page 124) will give you about 20g of carbohydrate. When you accompany this with a wholemeal roll, a green salad and a portion of fruit, you have an ideal meal containing three to four portions (about 60g) of carbohydrate. The addition of a bowl of beef and bean soup (see recipe, page 74) will increase this to five portions (about 75g) of carbohydrate.

Of course, your carbohydrate intake can be made up of half portions or double portions, depending on what suits you. Remember, the figures are only approximate, and you don't have to be precise. Generally, we do not recommend snacking between meals for overweight, less active people. If you are young, active or involved in vigorous exercise, or if your medications make it necessary, you may need to include high-carbohydrate snacks in your eating plan. But remember, snacking can contribute unnecessary calories which, in turn, can lead to weight gain.

Below we have a simple meal plan which shows you how to put into practice the information we give. The carbohydrate-rich foods have been highlighted for easy identification. The quantities of food will vary from person to person, and your weight is the best guide. This menu is, of course, rather plain, but it does show how to distribute your carbohydrate evenly through the day.

BREAKFAST	LUNCH	DINNER	BEDTIME SNACK
1 serving **wholegrain cereal** with low-fat milk 1 piece **fruit** 1–2 slices **wholemeal toast** or **granary bread** with reduced-fat spread and a topping of your choice	2 slices **wholemeal** or **granary bread** or **bread roll** with reduced-fat spread 1 thin slice of lean red meat or chicken (no skin) or tuna or salmon or egg or low-fat cheese plenty of salad vegetables 1–2 pieces of **fruit**	1 small portion lean red or white meat or fish 2 portions **starchy vegetables** or **pasta** or **rice** plenty of non-starchy vegetables 1 piece **fruit** and/or **low-fat yoghurt**	1 slice **wholemeal** or **granary bread** (with a scrape of reduced-fat spread) or **wholemeal biscuit**, and/or 1 mug low-fat milk as drink

MEAL PLANS

You know your approximate energy requirements, and roughly how much of each of the major nutrients you need daily. You also know that you should spread your carbohydrate through the day.

So far we have talked about nutrients. The following pages show you how to adapt this information and relate it to actual foods, rather than nutrients, ie. theory into practice. We have included four different examples of daily energy needs. Most men will require approximately 2500 kcal/day and for most women, 2000 kcal/day. The lower daily intakes may be appropriate for helping with weight loss, but please discuss your individual needs with your dietician first.

Sample meal plans

Water, tea, coffee or other low calorie beverage may be drunk with or between meals as desired.

Approx. 1500 kcal

BREAKFAST
- 2 wheat bisks served with 200ml (third of a pint) semi-skimmed milk
- 1 glass unsweetened fruit juice

MID MORNING
- 1 piece of fruit

LUNCH
- 1 sandwich made with 2 slices wholemeal or granary bread (or large roll) with low-fat spread and filled with 30g (1½oz) cheddar cheese and salad
- 1 piece of fruit

MID AFTERNOON
- fruit

EVENING MEAL
- Orange Borscht Soup
- 1 portion Meatballs in Tomato Sauce with rice
- 1 portion Vegetables Julienne
- 1 portion Mocha Mousse

- 200ml semi-skimmed milk included for use in drinks

NUTRITION INFORMATION
Energy & Nutrients: 1479 kcal; 63g protein; 49g fat; 194g carbohydrate (CHO)
Energy Ratio: 17% protein; 30% fat; 53% CHO

Approx. 1800 kcal

BREAKFAST
- 2 wheat bisks served with 200ml (third of a pint) semi-skimmed milk
- 1 glass unsweetened fruit juice
- 1 slice wholemeal toast spread with mono/polyunsaturated spread and marmalade

MID MORNING
- 1 piece of fruit

LUNCH
- 1 sandwich made with 2 slices wholemeal or granary bread (or large roll) spread with mono/poly spread and filled with 30g (1½oz) cheddar cheese and salad
- 1 piece of fruit

MID AFTERNOON
- fruit

EVENING MEAL
- Orange Borscht Soup
- 1 portion Meatballs in Tomato Sauce with rice
- 1 portion Vegetables Julienne
- 1 portion Mocha Mousse

- 200ml semi-skimmed milk included for use in drinks

NUTRITION INFORMATION
Energy & Nutrients: 1802 kcal; 66g protein; 66g fat; 236g CHO
Energy Ratio: 15% protein; 33% fat; 52% CHO

Sample meal plans

Water, tea, coffee or other low calorie beverage may be drunk with or between meals as desired.

Approx. 2000 kcal

BREAKFAST
- 2 wheat bisks served with 200ml (third of a pint) semi-skimmed milk
- I glass unsweetened fruit juice
- I slice wholemeal toast spread with mono/poly spread and marmalade

MID MORNING
- I piece of fruit

LUNCH
- I sandwich made with 2 slices wholemeal or granary bread (or large roll) spread with low-fat spread and filled with 30g (1½oz) cheddar cheese and salad
- 30g bag reduced fat crisps
- I piece of fruit

MID AFTERNOON
- I toasted crumpet spread with mono/poly spread and reduced sugar jam

EVENING MEAL
- Orange Borscht Soup
- I portion Meatballs in Tomato Sauce with rice
- I portion Vegetables Julienne
- I portion Mocha Mousse

- 200ml semi-skimmed milk included for use in drinks

NUTRITION INFORMATION
Energy & Nutrients: 2058 kcal; 70g protein; 79g fat; 270g CHO
Energy Ratio: 14% protein; 34% fat; 52% CHO

Approx. 2500 cal

BREAKFAST
- 2 wheat bisks served with 200ml (third of a pint) semi-skimmed milk
- I glass unsweetened fruit juice
- 2 slice wholemeal toast spread with mono/poly spread and marmalade

MID MORNING
- I piece of fruit
- I digestive biscuit

LUNCH
- I sandwich made with 2 slices wholemeal or granary bread (or large roll) spread with mono/poly spread and filled with 30g (1½oz) cheddar cheese and salad
- 30g bag reduced fat crisps
- I piece of fruit

MID AFTERNOON
- I toasted crumpet spread with low fat spread and reduced sugar jam
- fruit

DINNER
- Orange Borscht Soup
- I portion Meatballs in Tomato Sauce with rice
- I portion Vegetables Julienne
- I wholemeal/granary roll with mono/poly spread
- I portion Mocha Mousse

SUPPER/SNACK
- low fat fruit yoghurt

- 200ml semi-skimmed milk included for use in drinks

NUTRITION INFORMATION
Energy & Nutrients: 2460 kcal; 81g protein; 92g fat; 331g CHO
Energy Ratio: 13% protein; 33% fat; 54% CHO

Sample vegetarian meal plans

Water, tea, coffee or other low calorie beverage may be drunk with or between meals as desired.

Approx. 1500 kcal

BREAKFAST
- 2 wheat bisks served with 200ml (third of a pint) semi-skimmed milk
- 150ml glass unsweetened orange juice

MID MORNING
- 1 piece of fruit

LUNCH
- 1 sandwich made with 2 slices wholemeal/granary bread with low-fat spread, peanut butter and salad (eg. chopped celery and lettuce)
- 1 piece of fruit

MID AFTERNOON
- fruit

EVENING MEAL
- Orange Borscht Soup (made with vegetable stock)
- 1 portion Jumping Bean Bake
- 1 portion tossed salad
- 1 portion Mocha Mousse

NUTRITION INFORMATION
Energy & Nutrients: 1519 kcal; 81g protein; 48g fat; 206g carbohydrate (CHO)
Energy Ratio: 21% protein; 28% fat; 54% CHO

Approx. 1800 kcal

BREAKFAST
- 2 wheat bisks served with 200ml (third of a pint) semi-skimmed milk
- 150ml glass unsweetened orange juice
- 1 slice wholemeal toast with mono/poly spread and marmalade

MID MORNING
- 1 piece of fruit
- 1 plain digestive biscuit

LUNCH
- 1 sandwich made with 2 slices wholemeal/granary bread with mono/poly spread, peanut butter and salad (eg. chopped celery and lettuce)
- 1 piece of fruit

MID AFTERNOON
- fruit

EVENING MEAL
- Orange Borscht Soup (made with vegetable stock)
- 1 portion Jumping Bean Bake
- 1 portion tossed salad
- 1 portion Mocha Mousse

SUPPER/SNACK
- 1 toasted crumpet with reduced sugar jam

- 200ml semi-skimmed milk included for use in drinks

NUTRITION INFORMATION
Energy & Nutrients: 1844 kcal; 80g protein; 60g fat; 249g CHO
Energy Ratio: 17% protein; 29% fat; 54% CHO

Sample vegetarian meal plans

Water, tea, coffee or other low calorie beverage may be drunk with or between meals as desired.

Approx. 2000 kcal

BREAKFAST
- 2 wheat bisks served with 200ml (third of a pint) semi-skimmed milk
- 150ml glass unsweetened orange juice
- 1 slice wholemeal toast with mono/poly spread and marmalade

MID MORNING
- 1 piece of fruit
- 1 plain digestive biscuit

LUNCH
- 1 sandwich made with 2 slices wholemeal/granary bread with mono/poly spread, peanut butter and salad (eg. chopped celery and lettuce)
- 30g bag reduced fat crisps
- 2 pieces of fruit

MID AFTERNOON
- 1 toasted crumpet with reduced sugar jam

EVENING MEAL
- Orange Borscht Soup (made with vegetable stock)
- 1 portion Jumping Bean Bake
- 1 portion tossed salad
- 1 portion Mocha Mousse

SUPPER/SNACK
- 1 sandwich with 1 slice wholemeal/granary bread spread with mono/poly spread and yeast extract/salad

- 200ml skimmed milk included for use in drinks

NUTRITION INFORMATION
Energy & Nutrients: 2097 kcal; 91g protein; 71g fat; 285g CHO
Energy Ratio: 16% protein; 30% fat; 54% CHO

Approx. 2500 kcal

BREAKFAST
- 2 wheat bisks served with 200ml (third of a pint) semi-skimmed milk
- 150ml glass unsweetened orange juice
- 2 slices wholemeal toast with mono/poly spread and marmalade

MID MORNING
- 1 piece of fruit
- 1 plain digestive biscuit

LUNCH
- 1 sandwich made with 2 slices wholemeal/granary bread with low-fat spread, peanut butter and salad (eg. chopped celery and lettuce)
- 30g bag reduced fat crisps
- 2 pieces of fruit

MID AFTERNOON
- 1 toasted crumpet with mono/poly spread and reduced sugar jam

EVENING MEAL
- Orange Borscht Soup (made with vegetable stock)
- 1 portion Jumping Bean Bake
- 1 wholemeal roll with mono/poly spread
- 1 portion tossed salad
- 1 portion Mocha Mousse

SUPPER/SNACK
- 1 sandwich with 1 slice wholemeal/granary bread spread with mono/poly spread and yeast extract/salad

- 200ml skimmed milk included for use in drinks

NUTRITION INFORMATION
Energy & Nutrients: 2440 kcal; 95g protein; 93g fat; 315g CHO
Energy Ratio: 15% protein; 34% fat; 51% CHO

TIMING YOUR MEALS

To help you control your blood glucose level, you should eat regular meals.

If you're not on medication, in most cases spreading your carbohydrate evenly between three meals a day is best. Make sure that you have three to four servings of high-carbohydrate foods per meal, eg. 3 potatoes, a piece of fruit etc., but the punctuality of mealtimes is not as important as it would be if you were on medication, since you will not be prone to low blood glucose (hypoglycaemia). Avoid eating snacks between meals if you are overweight.

If you're on insulin or diabetes tablets, then you need to ask what type and when to take it. These questions are best answered in conjunction with your doctor, diabetes nurse and/or dietitian. Find out about your medication so that you can design an eating plan that allows your carbohydrate to be spread in such a way as to keep your blood glucose level within normal range. An even spread of carbohydrate between three meals daily is usually best, although some people find it easier to regulate blood glucose levels if they eat a carbohydrate-rich snack between meals. You may find that leaving long gaps between meals, or not eating enough carbohydrate at a meal, may cause your blood glucose level to drop too low (we discuss low blood glucose, hypoglycaemia, on page 39). It is also important to keep your carbohydrate intake even from day to day to prevent unwanted swings in blood glucose level.

Remember, having diabetes does not affect your need for energy, carbohydrate, protein and fat. It only affects the timing and planning of your meals. On the other hand, your meals and meal pattern must suit your lifestyle, and it may be easier to change the timing and dose of your medication rather than your established eating pattern.

INJECTED INSULIN AND MEALS

There are various types of insulin available, classified as short-, medium-, long-acting, or a combination of these depending on when their activity peaks, and the length of action. Short-acting insulins start to lower your blood glucose level immediately after injection; medium and long-acting insulins may take several hours to begin, and then continue to lower your blood glucose level for several more hours. The time you eat your carbohydrate should match the activity of your insulin. Discuss with your doctor, diabetes nurse or dietitian.

It is common for people with Type 1 diabetes to have an injection of short-acting insulin with each meal. This reflects the body's normal response to eating meals, where insulin levels in the blood increase as the carbohydrate (sugar and starches) is absorbed as glucose. This allows the opportunity to adjust food intake to suit daily lifestyle changes. A long-acting insulin is given prior to bed and helps control the blood glucose levels overnight.

EATING OUT

Having diabetes does not mean you have to miss out on the good things in life, such as eating out. What it does mean is that you need to understand your diabetes and how to manage it so that you can live the way you want to. Armed with this book and a bit of practice, you will build up the necessary confidence.

Finding your way around the menu

Meals out don't have to be dull and a few simple changes can make the menu offered at most restaurants fit your needs. The waiter can tell you what is in dishes if you are unsure. Don't be afraid to ask for meals to be prepared with minimal fat and for dressings and sauces to be served separately.

Because restaurant foods may be high in calories, you would be wise to limit yourself to a starter and main course, or to a main course and dessert.

The many restaurants offering wide-ranging types of cuisine are good choices. The following ideas may get you started:

- Italian: minestrone soup, pasta with a seafood or tomato sauce, salad, crusty bread, fruit platter or ice cream.
- Chinese: short soup, combination of seafood or meat and vegetables or whole fish in ginger, steamed vegetables, and steamed rice.
- Greek: dolmades, souvlaki, tabbouleh or Greek salad, plain pitta bread.
- Mexican: taco or burritos, green salad with salsa, refried beans, plain tortillas.
- Indian: tandoori chicken or fish, raita, vegetable curry, chappatis, steamed rice.
- Japanese: miso soup, sushi, nori or California rolls.
- Thai: clear soup with noodles, steamed rolls, salads or plain vegetables, and meat/fish dishes.

Soups

Thickened and 'creamed' soups will give you carbohydrate, but may be high in fats too. Ask the waiter to leave out the cream, or ask for a clear soup or a minestrone.

Entrées (starters)

Good choices are vegetable parcels, skewered meats, seafood on rice, simple salads, melon or other fruit-based dishes, smoked salmon, asparagus spears or pasta with vegetable sauce.

Main courses

Select small servings of lean chicken, fish, meat or seafood. Vegetarian and pasta dishes are fine, provided they are not loaded with cream, butter or cheese. To accompany your main course choose pasta, potato or rice to give you plenty of carbohydrate, and other vegetables and salads to add variety, flavour and colour.

Bread

If the meal you choose does not contain enough carbohydrate, ask for extra bread, but try to avoid high-fat garlic or herbed breads.

Desserts

These are often high in fat, and may contain more sugar than is desirable. If you do like to have a sweet, ask for fruit, a simple fruit dessert, a crème caramel, hot soufflé, or fruit crumble served without cream or rich sauces.

Beverages
Limit your alcohol intake and don't be afraid to ask for a jug of iced water.

Take-away meals
These are often high in fat and salt. The following are better choices in terms of less fat:
- sandwiches, rolls or filled pita bread, hamburger (plain meat and salad), souvlaki, barbecued or char-grilled chicken (no skin), steamed dim sum, hot dog, wholemeal pastie, jacket potatoes (without the sour cream).
- where possible, order some fresh salad or fruit to balance the meal.

TREATS AND SPECIAL OCCASIONS

Religious or feast days, birthdays and other family get-togethers are especially tempting. If you are the host, choose special recipes from this book for just such occasions. If you are a guest, have a little of the dishes you like, but balance this with vegetables, salad, bread and fruit.

A splurge now and then, on special occasions, does no harm; it's what you do for the rest of the time that counts. Return to your usual eating pattern at the next meal. Frequent splurging will contribute to weight gain and poorly controlled diabetes.

TRAVEL

When travelling short distances, try to have your meals at the normal times. When travelling by car, carry dry biscuits and fresh or dried fruits to eat if there are delays.

Overseas travel may mean a change in your normal pattern, particularly when you travel quickly across time zones. It is advisable to notify the airline well in advance and request additional fresh fruit, breads, sandwiches and dry biscuits.

If you are going to cross time zones, discuss your insulin and food requirements with your doctor, dietitian or diabetes nurse before you leave on the trip. When travelling in different countries, you can always find suitable food even if it is limited in variety.

SHIFT WORK

If you are a shift worker, the timing of your meals and medications may vary with the timing of your shifts. Because of the great variation in shifts and individual needs, it is difficult to give suggestions other than to strongly advise you to see a dietitian or diabetes nurse for help. Basically you should aim to spread your meals and diabetes medication throughout your waking hours, just as you would on day shift—and treat the day as night. Make sure, if you take your medication prior to going to bed, that you have also eaten.

SPECIAL NEEDS

HYPOGLYCAEMIA

When your blood glucose level drops too low, this is known as hypoglycaemia or a 'hypo'. Hypoglycaemia is defined as a blood glucose level below 3.5 mmol/l, and can happen to you if you are on insulin or diabetes tablets. It does not happen if you are being treated by diet alone.

How to recognise hypoglycaemia

The symptoms set in quickly. You may experience one or more of the following:
- headache
- dizziness, vagueness
- extreme hunger
- blurred vision
- sweating
- pins and needles around the mouth
- paleness, trembling, shaking
- drowsiness
- behaviour changes or mood swings (such as bad temper, crying, aggressiveness).

These signs tell you that your blood glucose level may have dropped too low. Some people who test their blood glucose level regularly may find that their level drops too low without experiencing any symptoms. If your blood glucose level drops below 3.5 mmol/l, it should be treated as hypoglycaemia whether you have symptoms or not.

What you should do if you have hypoglycaemia

1. Immediately take sugar to raise your blood glucose level. Any form of sugar will do but the following are recommended as they are absorbed quickly. Do not use low-calorie soft drinks to treat hypoglycaemia.
- A sweetened soft drink or Lucozade™—one glass.
- Confectionary such as jelly beans.
- Sugar in water—about 3 teaspoons in a cup of water.
- Honey or jam—about 1 tablespoon.

2. If the symptoms don't improve in five minutes, or become worse, take more sugar as above.

3. If still no improvement in ten minutes, contact your doctor or local hospital without delay.

4. Always follow the concentrated sugar with a snack of more complex carbohydrate such as fruit, bread, milk or biscuits, or have your next meal if it is due. This will help prevent your blood glucose level from falling again. Do not count any extra food taken to treat hypoglycaemia as part of your regular meal plan. Continue with your usual meals.

If not treated promptly and properly, hypoglycaemia can worsen and lead to unconsciousness. If this happens, others (family, friends, work mates) need to know what to do:

- roll the person onto their left side. Make sure the airway is clear, tilt the chin up and check the tongue hasn't rolled back;
- call a doctor or ambulance immediately;
- never give an unconscious person anything to eat or drink.

Medical treatment

The doctor will usually give an injection of a hormone called glucagon which stimulates the liver to release glucose into the bloodstream. Alternatively, he or she may inject a special glucose solution directly into the vein.

It is advisable to carry a small card containing the above information to assist others should you suffer a 'hypo' and become unconscious.

Why it happens

- Taking too much insulin.
- A meal delayed too long.
- Not enough carbohydrate in your food.
- Extra activity (without having extra carbohydrate foods to supply the extra energy—exercise uses your blood glucose supplies).
- Excess alcohol without carbohydrate—such as drinking whisky on an empty stomach.

Simple precautions to prevent hypoglycaemia

- Check your food intake to make sure you are having enough carbohydrate with each meal. If meals are delayed, have some carbohydrate in the form of a snack to tide you over.
- Check your dose of insulin or tablets carefully. Taking too much can make your blood glucose level fall too low.
- If you are more active than usual, you may need extra carbohydrate before, during and after the activity (see 'exercise, sport and diabetes', page 47).
- If you are drinking alcohol, make sure you eat food containing carbohydrate with it.

IMPORTANT: If you are having 'hypos' often, consult your doctor to discuss possible causes and solutions. If your diabetes is well controlled, you shouldn't have frequent 'hypos'.

WHAT TO DO IF YOU ARE ILL

If your diabetes is controlled without medication, don't worry if you are unable to eat properly for a day or two. Eat and drink as desired. If you are unwell for longer than this, discuss it with your doctor.

If you are on insulin or diabetes tablets, you must continue with your medication as usual, no matter how awful you are feeling. One of the side effects of various illnesses is that your blood glucose level rises, so your medications are absolutely vital to control this. Equally importantly, you must keep on taking carbohydrate even if you are off your food. To do this, try light meals, drinks high in carbohydrate or high-carbohydrate snacks. You may find it easier to have a snack or drink every hour, rather than attempt your usual daily meal pattern.

If you are ill for more than two days, or if your blood glucose is consistently higher than 15 mmol/litre, contact your doctor. The following are easy sources of carbohydrate if you are on medication:

- homemade or canned soup with toast or dry crackers
- plain boiled rice or noodles
- toast or sandwich
- dry crackers plain or with thinly sliced cheese, tomato or yeast extract
- lemonade or other soft drink, eg. diluted fruit squash
- jelly
- junket
- yoghurt, custard
- creamy rice
- plain sweet biscuit or cake
- stewed or canned fruit (in fruit juice)
- ice-cream
- milky drinks such as malted milk drinks
- fruit juice.

If nauseous or vomiting, try sipping drinks such as lemonade, diluted fruit squash or Lucozade™. Once you can tolerate any of these, nibble on a dry biscuit or toast, sip chicken noodle soup or try diluted apple or orange juice.

VOMITING OR DIARRHOEA

If you are vomiting or suffering from diarrhoea, be aware that it can lead to dehydration and uncontrolled diabetes. You need urgent treatment so contact your doctor right away.

HIGH BLOOD PRESSURE

Many people with high blood pressure can help bring it down by limiting the amount of salt (sodium) in their diet. If overweight, try to reduce your weight as another means of controlling your blood pressure.

If you have high blood pressure you would be wise to:

- limit the amount of salt you use in cooking;
- avoid adding salt at the table;
- limit the amount of highly salted processed food you eat.

Here is a list of some of the flavouring agents and processed foods which are high in salt:

- rock, sea and other salts—all of them are salt, no matter what the name;
- meat and vegetable extracts, stock cubes, stock powders and packet soups;
- salted, smoked, cured or pickled meat and fish;
- pickles, chutneys, relishes and dressings;
- canned meat, fish and vegetables;
- salted snacks, including potato and corn crisps, nuts and salted biscuits;
- take-away foods such as pizza, barbecued chicken.

Salt substitutes replace all or part of the sodium chloride with potassium chloride. Used sparingly these are a satisfactory substitute for ordinary salt, but it's probably best to train your taste buds to enjoy lower salt foods. It is wise to check with your doctor before using these substitutes.

There are many food products which are salt-reduced, such as breads, fat spreads and sauces. Use them in place of the salted varieties and check labels. Look out for the words sodium and salt. The sodium figure is listed in the nutrition panel. This will give an indication of salt level.

Another way in which to give your food zest without using added salt is through herbs and spices. Try adding lemon juice, tomato, onion, garlic or vinegar for extra flavour.

HIGH BLOOD FAT LEVELS (CHOLESTEROL AND TRIGLYCERIDES)

People who have high blood fat levels have an increased risk of heart and blood vessel disease. You run this risk regardless of whether you are overweight or of a healthy weight. The blood fats of concern are cholesterol and triglycerides. Both of these fats are made in the body as well as being provided in foods.

Cholesterol is found only in animal products, while triglycerides are found in both animal and vegetable foods. Foods high in cholesterol include egg yolk, liver, prawns, squid and fish roe.

Ninety-six per cent of fat in the diet is in the form of triglycerides. These fats can be categorised as saturated, monounsaturated or polyunsaturated according to their chemical structure. Animal fats are high in saturated fats which may cause a rise in blood cholestorol levels and contribute to heart disease. Saturated fats are found in fatty cuts of meat, full fat dairy products, butter, cakes, biscuits, savoury snacks and confectionery. Vegetable fats/oils tend to be higher in monounsaturated and polyunsaturated fats which protect against heart disease. Monounsaturated fats are found mainly in olive and rapeseed oils and spreads made from these. Polyunsaturated fats are found in pure vegetable oils, spreads made from these, seeds and nuts.

All fats have the same amount of calories per gram. Polyunsaturated and monounsaturated oils and spreads are still high in fats (apart from low-fat spreads). All fats should be used sparingly, particularly if you are trying to manage your weight. Although an intake of foods high in fat may increase triglyceride levels, this level can also be raised by alcohol. High triglyceride levels may also be found in overweight people and in people with undiagnosed or poorly controlled diabetes. Weight loss and establishing good control of diabetes will help reduce these levels.

Generally, limit all fats and, in particular, saturated fats in your diet. See page 18 for hints to help you use less fat. If you are concerned about the amount of fat in your diet or require greater detail on the types of fats, talk to your dietician.

PREGNANCY AND DIABETES

Diabetes should not stand in the way of a normal, healthy pregnancy. If you have diabetes, make sure that it is under good control where possible before you become pregnant. You will find that both your nutritional needs and your insulin dosage may need changing while you are pregnant. Get expert help from a dietitian and diabetes specialist and have your diabetes reviewed frequently during your pregnancy so your baby gets the best possible start and you maintain your health throughout.

You may also need to change the timing of your carbohydrate intake at this time, to help with management of your diabetes. It is particularly important that you eat regular meals, especially breakfast and a bedtime snack. Long periods without food may increase your risk of ketosis which can be harmful to you and to your baby. A general recommendation during pregnancy is to use artificial sweeteners sparingly and to avoid products sweetened with saccharin and cyclamates (see pages 26–28 for information on other artificial sweeteners).

Developing diabetes while pregnant (gestational diabetes)

Some women develop diabetes for the first time during pregnancy, usually after the twenty-sixth week. Once the baby is born, the symptoms may disappear, and reappear in later pregnancies. It is quite common for women who develop gestational diabetes to develop Type 2 diabetes later in life.

To ensure that you and your baby are healthy, once you have been diagnosed as having diabetes, you must take particular care of your diet throughout the remainder of your pregnancy. Medication is frequently necessary to ensure good blood glucose control.

Furthermore, if you control your weight from then on, exercise regularly and make sure your diet is well balanced with plenty of starchy, high-fibre foods and fruit and vegetables, you can help delay the onset of diabetes in later life. This underlines an important point: good nutrition and keeping a healthy weight are two of your best protections against developing diabetes.

CHILDREN AND ADOLESCENTS

You will find the guidelines set out in this book will ensure that children and adolescents with diabetes enjoy the benefits of up-to-date dietary management.

Just as their insulin requirements will vary, so will their dietary needs; it is a good idea to have your child or adolescent's diet reviewed at least annually by a dietitian, and their diabetes and general health monitored regularly. However, do remember that for all children food has important social implications. While encouraging enjoyment of a healthy eating plan, you may have to compromise at times. Food and eating should not become a battlefield, a focus of rebellion or a source of family tension. To begin with, the entire family would benefit by eating in exactly the same way. This takes away any sense of 'being different' or feeling deprived.

There is a common misconception that the food you should prepare for your offspring with diabetes is by its very nature unpalatable and 'unusual'. The menu plans and recipes in this book show just how unnecessary and wrong this view is; teach all your children about a varied and balanced eating plan, encourage a liking for cereals, vegetables and fruit, and you will have achieved something of lifelong value.

Be flexible and make an effort in the kitchen to prepare food that delights and satisfies. Remember, too, that children and adolescents like to snack, so prepare healthy and delicious ones in advance so that you don't hear the complaint, 'There's nothing to eat', meaning, 'There is nothing ready prepared which I can pick up in my fingers right away'. This avoids problems where children and adolescents turn to fast foods and processed products because they are so easy to get hold of. Providing alternatives is half the battle; good sense will see you through the rest.

Tips and traps for children and adolescents

- With young children, it is important that they take an active part in their diabetes management, including blood glucose monitoring, their insulin injections, food choices and planning their meals. You will find that the more involved your child is, the less tension is likely to arise.
- Avoid making diabetes the focus of family life—it's just one aspect. Don't force your child to eat; you don't always feel hungry and neither do they. Forcing a reluctant child to eat leads to resentment, rebellion and anxiety for everyone. It's totally counter-productive. You may find, in the name of co-operation and family well-being, that you have to sometimes make a temporary compromise on diabetes control for the sake of the long-term outcome.
- By learning to monitor their own blood glucose level, your child will soon learn the effects different foods have on it.

- Teach your children the benefits of regular meals and a healthy way of eating. It's an investment in their future health. Use this approach and your child will come to see healthy eating as a positive aspect of life rather than as a negative aspect of having diabetes. Children (and adults for that matter) should learn that diabetes does not mean being punished or deprived of food.
- It's easy to fall into the trap of replacing uneaten vegetables and cereals with sugary foods because of a fear of hypoglycaemia. Children are smart and they will soon learn to manipulate; they may start refusing their meals knowing you may offer them a sweet treat instead. Try offering healthier alternatives in this situation: fruit, milk or wholegrain bread will do the trick.
- Encourage your child to carry extra snacks, especially when they will be away from home for long periods such as sleeping out on weekends or going to after-school activities.
- Make sure parents of friends, and teachers at school, know that your child has diabetes and that they know how to cope with hypoglycaemia and sickness.
- Let your child know that there are other children with diabetes. They are neither alone nor unique. Diabetes camps are an excellent way to reduce any sense of isolation. Your local hospital, dietician or diabetes nurse will have details.
- Diabetes is not a barrier to normal childhood activities such as parties, sport, staying at friends', trips or school camps, and you should encourage your child to take part.
- The better your child understands his or her diabetes, the more responsibility they will take for it and so they will cope better with their own changing needs as they grow older.
- Don't turn your child into a 'cupboard cater' or 'food sneak' by never letting them taste sweet foods. That old phrase, 'moderation in all things' holds good. You may well find that denying your child any sweet foods leads to secret eating and binges. Simply try not to make a fuss about fatty or sweet foods; remember that the occasional splurge will not cause any long-term harm.
- Adolescence brings its own special needs. The teens are a time of exploration, testing and a desire or need for independence. This applies to the issue of food just as much as it does to other realms of behaviour. If your teenager has a good knowledge of diabetes management, they will know how to be flexible in terms of mealtimes, foods eaten, the amount of insulin they need and when they need it. This may cause you considerable anxiety, but it's important to learn to encourage your child's sense of independence; allow them to learn by their own mistakes.
- For adolescents, the peer pressure to drink alcohol may be strong. Make sure your teenager understands how vital it is for them to have plenty of carbohydrate when they drink alcohol.
- Adolescents also need to realise how vital it is to seek medical help the moment they do not feel well. Failure to do this is a common cause of hospital admissions for uncontrolled diabetes.
- Hormonal changes and growth spurts during adolescence may upset your adolescents' diabetes control even though they are doing the right thing. It may be that their whole management routine needs a fresh appraisal.

VEGETARIANS WITH DIABETES

The guidelines in this book are ideal for people who are vegetarian. Many of the recipes have been created with vegetarians in mind, and on pages 34–35 you will find vegetarian meal plans showing how to balance your nutritional needs.

You can follow a vegetarian diet, be well nourished and keep your diabetes under control. But you should to be aware that as a vegetarian you can miss out on some nutrients. It is therefore vital that you know how to plan your diet to ensure these are included in adequate amounts.

To begin with, we suggest that you include dairy products and eggs in your vegetarian eating plan (in other words, what is termed 'lacto-ovo vegetarian'). However, if you choose out of matters of conscience or religion to follow a strict vegan lifestyle (in other words, you do not eat any animal products at all), we strongly recommend that you consult a dietitian, who will help you plan a nutritionally balanced diet. The principles in this book apply to vegetarians; however, there are other tips which are particularly important.

Tips and traps for vegetarians
- The nutrients that may be lacking in a poorly planned diet are: iron, zinc, protein, calcium, cyanocobalamin (Vitamin B12) and riboflavin (B2).
- The best sources of iron and zinc for vegetarians are pulses, wholegrain cereal products, green leafy vegetables and eggs. However, these foods do not release their minerals into your system as readily as do animal sources, such as meat.
- To increase your absorption of iron from non-meat sources, include foods with Vitamin C at the same meal. For instance, include citrus fruits, pineapple, tomatoes or juice made from them when you eat iron-rich food such as cereal products, spinach or silverbeet.
- The tannin in tea interferes with the absorption of iron into your body, so try not to finish your meal with a cup of tea.
- Fibre slows the absorption of vitamins and minerals in your digestive tract, so you may have to eat more of certain foods to counter this.
- Aim to eat the recommended daily amounts of dairy products and eggs set out below, to ensure your protein, calcium, cyanocobalamin (B12) and riboflavin (B2) needs are met.

Recommended daily food intake for lacto-ovo vegetarians
Milk and dairy products
600ml (1 pint) milk or the equivalent in cheese and/or yoghurt.
- 200ml milk = 30g hard cheese = 1 carton (150g) yoghurt

NOTE: Low-fat cheeses such as cottage and ricotta are not such good sources of calcium. Low-fat milk provides a little more calcium than whole milk.

Other protein-rich foods
We recommend that you eat two portions of the following every day:

- eggs: 1 portion = 2 eggs
- pulses: 1 portion = 150g (5oz)
- nuts: 1 portion = 90g

NOTE: Because vegetarian diets are generally low in high cholesterol foods, don't worry about limiting your intake of eggs.

Guidelines for other foods

Make sure that your daily diet also includes:

- 5 or more servings of fruit and vegetables – all types;
- bread and cereals: eat to appetite, but include some with every meal;
- fats: small amounts of cooking oils/spreading fats.

Tips for vegans

- Suitable protein sources include calcium fortified soy milk, pulses, nuts, seeds and cereal products. As the protein quality from these sources is different to animal sources, you need to eat a variety of these products every day.
- Alternative cyanocobalamin (B12) sources include some fortified soy milk (check the label). As only a few milks are fortified, a supplement may be required.
- Alternative calcium sources include fortified soy milk (check the label). Sesame and sunflower seeds, tahine, almonds and dried apricots contain small amounts of calcium.
- Alternative riboflavin (B2) sources include fortified soy milk (check the label), yeast extract, dried fruits, pulses, nuts and green leafy vegetables.

A NOTE ABOUT SOY MILK AND DIABETES

Many brands of soy milk have added sugar. This is also common in flavoured soy milk, so check the labels. Unsweetened soy milks are poor sources of calcium, riboflavin (B2) and cyanocobalamin (B12), so you may need a supplement.

EXERCISE, SPORT AND DIABETES

Regular, moderate physical activity is important for everyone who wants to achieve and maintain good health. This means aiming for thirty minutes most days of the week. Choose an activity you enjoy such as brisk walking, swimming, cycling, dancing, gardening, golf, etc. 'Moderate' exercise means moving about enough to make you feel warm and slightly out of breath.

For people with diabetes, exercise has another function: it helps keep their blood glucose level within normal range. People with Type 2 diabetes can improve the control of their diabetes and minimise their need for medication by exercising or being physically active regularly.

If you have Type 1 diabetes, regular exercise is important, but requires more careful planning. You will learn from experience how your body reacts to exercise and how best to balance your energy expenditure with the needs of your diabetes.

Exercise and your blood glucose level

For the person without diabetes, the body is able to keep blood glucose level constant during sport through the release of insulin and other hormones. When exercise begins, the body normally stops releasing insulin and produces the hormones adrenalin and glucagon which stimulate the liver to release glucose into the blood. The insulin already present in the bloodstream allows the exercising muscles to take up the glucose, converting it to energy and keeping the blood glucose level constant.

As the exercise continues, the blood glucose level normally goes up and the liver then stops releasing glucose. Now the body releases insulin again, so that more glucose can pass into the exercising muscle. This complex mechanism ensures that the blood glucose level normally remains constant.

What happens if you have Type 1 diabetes?

If you have Type 1 diabetes, your body is not able to respond in the same way to exercise. Once you have taken your insulin injection, you cannot regulate its action. This means that you may have a wide variation in your blood glucose level during and after exercise. However, if you have enough insulin in your system and your blood glucose level is within the normal range at the start of exercise, then you can safely exercise.

If you don't have enough insulin available in your system when you begin exercising—in other words, your blood glucose level is high—your body can misread the situation and release more glucose into your bloodstream from the liver. Because you don't have enough insulin, the glucose can't pass into your muscle cells. As a result, your blood glucose level will rise excessively (hyperglycaemia). So check your glucose levels before you begin. You shouldn't exercise if your blood glucose is above 15 mmol/l.

If, on the other hand, you have too much insulin in your blood and your blood glucose level is low, your liver shuts down its release of glucose. The insulin continues to carry glucose to your muscles, leading to a rapid fall in your blood glucose level (hypoglycaemia). In this case take more carbohydrate before you begin to exercise.

Tips and traps

Hypoglycaemia is the most common concern for people on diabetes medication who exercise regularly. However, there are some simple steps you can take to help prevent this problem.

- Where possible, check your blood glucose level before you exercise, especially if you are new to diabetes. If your level is low, then take a carbohydrate snack before you begin exercising. You may find it useful to take another test after the exercise, or during it if it is prolonged, so you become familiar with the effect exercise has on your blood glucose level.
- If you are exercising away from home, make sure you have some carbohydrate foods with

you, such as fruit, fruit juice or biscuits.

- If you have been doing vigorous exercise, your blood glucose level may continue to drop after you stop exercising, so you should eat a carbohydrate-containing snack or meal afterwards, too.
- Be aware of dehydration. But don't confuse this with hypoglycaemia which relates not to fluids but to blood glucose level. Be well hydrated before you start exercise, top up during exercise and drink freely afterwards.
- When your exercise session is over, quench your thirst with a non-alcoholic drink, such as diluted fruit juice. Alcohol may lower your blood glucose level further and also has a dehydrating effect.
- Elite athletes with diabetes (and there are many) ensure that their diabetes is well controlled before they begin training. Training is the time to fine tune control. They know that this will ensure peak performance during competition.

ACTIVITY	TIME	BGL PRIOR TO ACTIVITY (mmol/l)	RECOMMENDED ADDITIONAL CARBOHYDRATE INTAKE
Low-level	1/2 hour	< 6	15g CHO (one portion fruit, bread, biscuit, yoghurt or milk).
		> 6	No extra food.
Moderate	1 hour	< 6	20–30g CHO (1½–2 portion fruit, bread, biscuits, yoghurt and/or milk).
		6–10	15g CHO (one portion fruit, bread, biscuit, yoghurt and/or milk).
		10–15	No extra food (in most cases).
		15	No extra food. Exercise not recommended: blood glucose level may go up.
Strenuous activity	1–2 hours	< 6	45–60g CHO (1 sandwich and fruit and /or milk or yoghurt).
		6–10	25–50g CHO (1 sandwich and fruit and/or milk or yoghurt).
		10–15	15g CHO (1 portion fruit, bread, biscuits, yoghurt or milk).
		> 15	Exercise not recommended: blood glucose level may go up.
Varying intensity	1/2 –1 day		Insulin may best be decreased. (Conservatively decrease the insulin dose due to peak at time of activity by 10 per cent. A 50 per cent reduction is not uncommon.)
CHO=Carbohydrate			Increase CHO before, during and after activity.
BGL=Blood Glucose Level			15–50g CHO per hour, such as diluted fruit juice, or sports drinks.

How to adjust your food intake

Once your diabetes is controlled, you will need to learn how to manipulate the balance between food, insulin and activity. The only way to do this properly is to monitor your blood glucose level before, during and after you exercise and experiment until you are confident about the combination which suits your needs best.

If you are a competitive athlete, you might want to talk to your dietician about your individual needs.

HOW TO MODIFY RECIPES

Some of your old favourite family recipes may seem unsuitable if you have diabetes. As we've mentioned already, when you have diabetes you don't have to eat special foods – a diet for diabetes is a healthy diet.

It can be quite easy to adapt a typical family dish to be healthier. We have made changes in ingredients and method to the dish below. These are shown in italics.

Bread and Butter Pudding

4 thin slices bread *use wholemeal bread*

2 tablespoons butter *3 teaspoons should be enough and use polyunsaturated margarine*

4 tablespoons sugar *use 1–2 tablespoons sugar or an alternative sweetener*

add vanilla essence for more flavour

½ cup raisins

2 eggs

600ml (1 pint) milk *use semi-skimmed milk*

1. Grease a pie dish. *No need to grease.*
2. Spread the bread with butter *(reduced-fat spread)* and layer it in the dish with sugar and raisins sprinkled in between. *Use less sugar, or if you prefer a sweet pudding, add sweetener to the eggs and milk.*
3. Beat the eggs and milk. *Add vanilla and sweetener if preferred to sugar.*
4. Pour egg mixture over the bread and leave to stand for 10 minutes. Then bake in moderate oven until the custard is set, approximately 20–25 minutes.

Tips and traps in modifying recipes

Main dishes

- Consider whether you can cut down on the amount of meat—50–75g (2–3oz) per person is sufficient. This means 300g should feed four.
- Choose lean cuts and trim off any visible fat.
- If bacon is used as a flavouring, trim off fat or use back bacon.
- Limit fats. For browning foods, use a non-stick pan to dry fry foods such as meat. Alternatively, use a cooking spray or a pastry brush to brush a thin layer of oil on the base of the pan—you really need very little to do the trick.
- When using oil, always measure it out in tablespoons rather than pouring it straight from the bottle. Try using less oil than the recipe suggests.
- If a recipe uses cream or sour cream as a sauce, you can often use low-fat yoghurt or fromage frais instead, but remember to add it at the last minute and not allow the sauce to

reboil or the yoghurt/fromage frais will curdle.

- For white sauces, use semi-skimmed or skimmed milk in place of full cream milk. You can use a low-fat spread if you cook the sauce in an all-in-one recipe. Alternatively use cornflour (cornstarch) with semi-skimmed milk to thicken sauces. You don't then need to use the fat.
- To add fibre and decrease the meat content of a dish, include some dried beans or lentils in mixed dishes with meat. This works wonderfully in pasta sauces, lasagne, curries and casseroles.

Desserts and cakes

Many of these recipes modify well, so try your old standbys with a few changes, such as:

- substitute wholemeal flour for white, or, if the result is too heavy, use a half-and-half mixture. If you substitute wholemeal flour in a recipe, you usually have to add a little more liquid to get a moist result;
- substitute margarine or reduced-fat spread for butter and substitute skimmed or semi-skimmed milk for full cream milk;
- where a recipe specifies that you cream butter (or margarine) and sugar, reduce the sugar, add butter (or margarine) and rub into the dry ingredients;
- where you have reduced butter and sugar in a recipe, it will not rise as high, and the texture will be a little denser. Try using a smaller baking tin.

And if your recipe can't be modified?...

Some recipes simply don't look and taste the same if modified. Put these on your list of occasional dishes and keep them as treats.

USING THE RECIPES IN THIS BOOK

Most of the recipes in this book are simple and quick to prepare. In most cases, we avoid using unusual ingredients, although we do slip some in to encourage you to experiment. Where a choice of ingredients is given in a recipe, the first one listed is the one we use in our analysis of nutritional value. The symbol ⏱ indicates the total preparation and cooking time needed for each recipe.

Flavour

You can increase or decrease the flavour intensity of recipes to suit your own taste. Experiment with herbs and spices; cut back or add more as you like. Such flavour-enhancers will not alter the nutritional value of your food.

If microwaving any of the dishes, you may need to increase the amount of herbs and spices we recommend because microwaving does not always allow for the flavours to develop and combine.

Salt

We follow the good health guideline for everyone to 'cut back on salt'. However, we use common sense, and where we feel that a recipe needs a little salt we add it or use soy sauce or stock cubes.

We encourage you to minimise or omit salt wherever possible. Where we refer to soy sauce in the recipes, we suggest you use light soy sauce.

Sugar

We use a variety of sweetening agents in our recipes, including sugar in small amounts. There are good reasons for this. Firstly, we now know that a small amount of sugar taken in a mixed meal or recipe does not cause a significant rise in the blood glucose level. Secondly, some recipes, especially baked products, rely on sugar to produce good results. Thirdly, there are some instances where the flavour of sugar is superior to that of artificial sweeteners—it does not alter or lose taste during the cooking process.

You will also see that we use natural sweetening agents other than sucrose (table sugar), such as fruit juice, dried fruits and fruit juice concentrates, with delicious results. A range of artificial sweeteners are also used.

Fat

We use a number of ways to reduce the fat content of our recipes. For example, we frequently sauté using water or a hot dry pan instead of oil. Where oil is used we have kept it to a minimum by recommending that you brush the frying pan with oil rather than pouring it in.

Generally, we use skimmed or semi-skimmed milk. Likewise, you can substitute low-fat natural yoghurt for whole milk yoghurt in most cases, but not always—for instance, whole milk yoghurt is absolutely necessary for quick wholemeal bread (see recipe page 203).

Where we use cottage cheese, it is always the skimmed milk variety; ricotta cheese is always low-fat ricotta; reduced-fat cheddar cheese is cheese of less than 17 per cent fat; and medium-fat soft cheese is the shop-bought variety of less than 17 per cent fat, or a homemade mixture of equal proportions of cottage cheese and cream cheese. To enhance the flavour of some recipes, we include a small amount of higher fat cheeses, such as parmesan. Here, we use the principle that a small amount goes a long way.

Fibre

We use wholemeal products as much as possible. However, there are times when the texture or flavour of the dish is better with a mixture of wholegrain and refined flours or cereals. In a few recipes, we use the refined product only to give a more traditional result. Using wholemeal flour products gives a heavier or denser texture than white flour, and requires more liquid during cooking. We allow for this in our recipes.

Using the oven

Always preheat your oven so it is at the correct temperature when you are ready to bake.

CHOOSING YOUR MEALS

1. Choose your carbohydrate: pasta, potato, rice, noodles, bread, couscous, polenta, legumes, cereals. Don't forget to include at least one carbohydrate food of low GI at each meal.
2. Consider your protein: meat, poultry, fish, seafoods, eggs, tofu, pulses/legumes, cheese, nuts.
3. Add plenty of vegetables and fruits, cooked or raw, as either the main part of a dish or as a side dish.
4. Choose your flavour. Traditionally, the UK diet has been rather plain and the flavours monotonous but over recent years the influence of other cultures, and in particular those of Asia and the Mediterranean, has encouraged us to add interest to our meals. The variety of herbs and spices and addition of garlic, onions, tomato and chilli is common.

TIME SAVER
- In a hurry? Try the assorted mixtures of vegetables from the freezer in your supermarket.
- Check the supermarket shelves or specialty grocers for pastes of chilli, garlic, ginger and shallots. There are also plenty of curry pastes, and packets, cans or jars of spices, pastes and sauces that offer a variety of different flavours. Check the food label and choose lower fat products whenever possible.

THINK TASTE, THINK FLAVOUR

Chinese
- sauces: chilli, hoisin, oyster, plum, soy • fresh/pastes: garlic, sesame, ginger, chilli • spices: five-spice, star anise • oils: chilli, sesame • other: onions, coriander, bamboo shoots, black beans, Chinese mushrooms, wood fungus, lily buds, lotus root, walnuts, spring onion, water chestnuts

Indian
- spices: cumin (seeds and ground), mustard seeds, black peppercorns, cardamom (pods and ground), cinnamon sticks, chilli powder, cloves (whole and ground), coriander (seeds and ground), curry leaves, fennel (seeds and ground), fenugreek (seeds and ground), garam masala, mace (ground), nutmeg (whole), saffron, tandoori mix, turmeric • other: onions, coconut milk (for a low-fat alternative mix 250ml reduced-fat, evaporated milk and ½ teaspoon coconut essence, or look for a commercial product with less than 6 per cent fat), ghee

Indonesian / Malaysian
- sauces: soy, sweet • fresh/pastes: chilli, shrimp • spices: coriander (ground), cumin (ground), tamarind, lemon grass, tumeric • oils: peanut, sesame • other: onions, coconut milk (or low-fat alternative), peanuts

Italian
- fresh/pastes: garlic • herbs: basil, oregano • other: onions, tomato, olives, anchovies, capers

Japanese

- sauces: Japanese soy, citrus soy • fresh/pastes: garlic, sesame, ginger, chilli • oils: sesame
- other: onion, spring onion

Thai

- sauces: light and dark soy, fish, chilli • herbs: coriander, mint • spices: black pepper, lemon grass, turmeric, dried chilli, ground cumin, ground coriander, paprika, whole and ground cinnamon, whole and ground cloves, cardamom pods, ground cardamom, tamarind • fresh/pastes: shrimp, garlic, sesame, ginger, chilli, tomato • oils: sesame, peanut • other: dried shrimps, raw peanuts, sesame seeds, onions, Chinese mushrooms, coconut milk or low-fat alternative), dried coconut, spring onion, rice wine or dry sherry, palm or dark brown sugar

BREAKFASTS

For a good start to a great day, make sure you have breakfast. We've given ideas from leisurely Sunday breakfasts through to simple quick ideas for the weekday rush. Breakfast can be as simple as a bowl of cereal and a serve of fruit, or as beguiling as a fruit platter followed by mouth-watering pancakes.

Start your day with plenty of carbohydrate and fibre. Begin with a breakfast cereal. This can be homemade or you can choose from the excellent commercial products available (see pages 208–209). Porridge makes a terrific start to the day and lends itself to interesting toppings such as sultanas, diced raw apple, cinnamon or nuts.

Make your own breakfast blend using oats, all-bran, wheatgerm, bran, dried fruits of every kind, unsalted raw nuts, seeds (pumpkin, sesame and sunflower), millet, buckwheat, puffed rice, wheat or corn and wheatflakes. Serve with hot or cold skimmed or semi-skimmed milk, yoghurt and fruit.

With toast or bread, look at the toppings and fillings suggested on page 61. Consider the recipes in this section for date and fig spread and dried apricot conserve.

Fruit cleanses the palate and provides vitamins and minerals as well as carbohydrate and fibre. Eat it fresh, stewed or canned without added sugar. Combine fruits, top them with low-fat yoghurt, cottage or ricotta cheese, or add them to porridge, cereal, or eat them on their own.

Cooked breakfasts are a pleasant treat. They need not take long to prepare. Try:

- baked beans with freshly chopped mushrooms or capsicum;
- tomatoes, asparagus, mushrooms or sweetcorn on toast;
- poached, scrambled or boiled eggs;
- omelettes, with fillings such as cheese and herbs, tomato combined with lean ham and onion, or a mushroom sauce.

MEG'S MUESLI

MAKES 1KG

- ◆ 4 cups rolled oats or barley
  (or 2 cups of each)
- ◆ 1 cup shredded coconut
- ◆ 1 cup sultanas
- ◆ 1 cup chopped unsalted cashews
  or almonds
- ◆ 2 cups barley or oat bran
- ◆ 2 cups all-bran
- ◆ 1½ cups wheatgerm

⏱ 15 minutes

You can develop your own muesli recipe according to taste, but be very careful about the ingredients you add—check them against the ready reckoner at the end of this book to find out whether the additional ingredients you want to use have more fat than we recommend. Watch out, too, for added sugar.

METHOD
1. Mix all ingredients well with a large spoon or your fingers.
2. Allow ⅓ cup per serving.

NUTRITION DATA PER SERVING:
112 kcal (470 kJ), CHO 12g, protein 4g, fat 6g.

LIQUID BREAKFAST

SERVES FOUR

- ◆ 2 cups (500ml) skim
  or low-fat milk
- ◆ 1 cup (250ml) low-fat
  natural yoghurt
- ◆ 3 ripe bananas or 1 cup (160g)
  fresh strawberries, unsweetened
  canned peaches or apricots
- ◆ 2 eggs (optional)
- ◆ Candarel™ or other artificial
  sweetener, to taste
- ◆ ground allspice, cinnamon or
  nutmeg, for garnish

⏱ 5 minutes

If you simply don't have a moment in the mornings, this quick breakfast comes in a glass.

METHOD
1. Place all ingredients in a blender or food processor and blend well.
2. Serve at once, topped with a sprinkling of spice.

NUTRITION DATA PER SERVING:
179 kcal (749 kJ), CHO 26g, protein 12g, fat 4g.

CODDLED EGG

SERVES ONE

- 1 egg
- 1 slice wholegrain bread
- ½ teaspoon margarine
- pepper and pinch of salt

⏱ 10 minutes

VARIATION: Add ½ teaspoon of finely chopped chives or parsley at step three.

METHOD

1. Bring water to boil in a saucepan, lower egg in gently and soft boil to preference (three to five minutes).
2. Crumble bread into an individual serving bowl.
3. Add margarine, pepper and salt.
4. Lift egg out of water, crack open top, and spoon soft egg onto bread mixture.
5. Stir together gently and serve.

NUTRITION DATA PER SERVING:
145 kcal (607 kJ), CHO 10g, protein 8g, fat 8g.

DATE AND FIG SPREAD

MAKES 2 CUPS (190g)

- 1 cup (210g) seedless dates
- 1 cup (210g) dried figs
- 6 teaspoons lemon juice
- ¼ cup (60ml) orange juice

⏱ 15 minutes plus overnight soaking

The dates and figs have all the sweetness you need as a substitute for traditional sugar-laden jams.

METHOD

1. Chop fruit finely.
2. Add to bowl, pour juice over, cover and soak overnight.
3. Spoon into blender or food processor and blend for approximately two minutes until smooth.
4. Store, covered, in a jar in the refrigerator for up to two weeks.

NUTRITION DATA PER TOTAL QUANTITY:
791 kcal (3312 kJ), CHO 196g, protein 10g, fat trace.

DRIED APRICOT CONSERVE

MAKES 1 CUP

- 1 cup (140g) dried apricots
- juice of 1 orange
- pinch of ground cloves
- ½ cup (125ml) warm water

⏱ 1½ hours

You can vary this delectable yet simple recipe by using a dried fruit medley, dried peaches or dried pears. You can also replace the cloves with fresh or ground ginger.

METHOD
1. Chop apricots roughly.
2. Combine in mixing bowl with juice, spices, and water. Cover. Allow to stand for one hour.
3. Spoon into saucepan and cook gently for approximately 10 minutes over low heat, stirring constantly, until mixture thickens and starts to combine. Alternatively, spoon into a bowl and microwave on high for five minutes. Stir two or three times during cooking until mixture thickens and starts to combine.
4. Spoon into container, cover and cool.
5. Stir again, adding a little more water if necessary, then refrigerate until ready to use for up to two weeks.

NUTRITION DATA PER TOTAL QUANTITY:
298 kcal (1248 kJ), CHO 69g, protein 8g, fat trace.

APPETISERS AND SNACKS

Here we give you some ideas for quick and light meals, parties and pre-dinner nibbles. Remember the basic principles of low fat when planning appetisers and snacks. The recipes in this section are also a useful source of carbohydrate. If you are trying to lose weight, be careful not to over-indulge in these tempting extras.

To start with, here are a few simple ideas:

ACCOMPANIMENTS FOR DIPS

Vegetables

• carrot sticks • cauliflower and broccoli florets • celery sticks • cucumber wedges • green or red capsicum (bell pepper) pieces • mushroom (button or slices) • radish wedges • spring onions

Fruit

• apple wedges tossed in lemon juice to prevent browning • melon (cantaloupe) or honey dew melon cut into chunks • kiwi fruit wedges • fresh pineapple pieces • pear slices • fresh apricot halves

Bread and biscuits

• crusty wholegrain bread • dark rye bread slices • triangles of toast • pitta bread triangles (fresh or toasted) • plain dry crispbread or savoury biscuits

LOW-FAT DIPS

French Onion

1. Spoon 125g low-fat Philadelphia cheese into a mixing bowl and beat until soft.
2. Add 125g smooth ricotta cheese or 100g low-fat natural yoghurt and mix well together.
3. Add half a packet of dried French onion soup mix and 1 tablespoon of chopped parsley or chives, and chill in the refrigerator until required.
4. Serve with bread sticks or vegetable sticks.

Tsatziki

1. Grate half an unpeeled cucumber into a colander and drain to remove as much water as possible. This is important otherwise the dip will be too watery.
2. Place in a mixing bowl and add 200g low-fat natural yoghurt, 1–2 cloves of crushed garlic, 2 teaspoons of chopped fresh mint or parsley, 1 tablespoon finely chopped spring onion and salt and pepper to taste.
3. Refrigerate until ready to serve.

Hummus

1. Drain and rinse one 400g can of chick peas.
2. Grind in a food processor or blender with 60ml lemon juice until smooth.
3. Add 1–2 teaspoons crushed garlic, 60ml tahini, salt and pepper to taste, a dash of paprika and 1 tablespoon chopped parsley (optional). Mix until well combined.
4. Serve with bread sticks, vegetable sticks or chunks of crusty bread.

PRAWN CRACKERS

1. Place a paper towel on the microwave turntable.
2. Place 8–10 prawn crackers on the towel, making sure they are separate.
3. Cook on high for 35–45 seconds, depending on the power level of the oven. (The crackers will puff up and become light and crisp, but take care not to overcook or they will burn.)
4. Serve alone as low fat 'nibbles', or with a dip.

POPPADUMS

1. Place a paper towel on the microwave turntable.
2. Place the dry poppadums on the paper, making sure they do not touch.
3. Cook on high for approximately 20 seconds, depending on the power level of the oven.
4. Serve with a dip of fruit chutney, fresh mango pickle, or raita (see recipes on pages 154, 172).

ASPARAGUS ROLLS

To serve four, you will need three slices of wholemeal bread and three slices of white high-fibre bread.
1. Cut off the crusts, roll the bread to flatten it a little, spread with margarine or reduced-fat mayonnaise very lightly.
2. Place a spear of cooked fresh asparagus or canned asparagus diagonally across each slice of bread. Roll the bread towards a corner, press lightly to seal the edges of the bread. Cut in half.
3. Garnish with rings of green or red capsicum (bell pepper) and parsley.

POTATO WEDGES

1. Preheat oven to 200°C.
2. Cut two medium potatoes, skin on, into wedges and steam or microwave until partly cooked.
3. Place in a large mixing bowl and add herbs and seasonings as desired.
4. Spray with a little spray oil, spread out on a baking sheet and bake until golden brown and crispy—about 30–45 minutes. Turn once during cooking period.
5. Serve with tomato-based salsa or a low-fat dip.

PUMPERNICKEL (RYE BREAD) SAVOURIES

Many different combinations can be used to top rounds or squares of pumpernickel to make interesting and tasty savouries. Try these ideas:

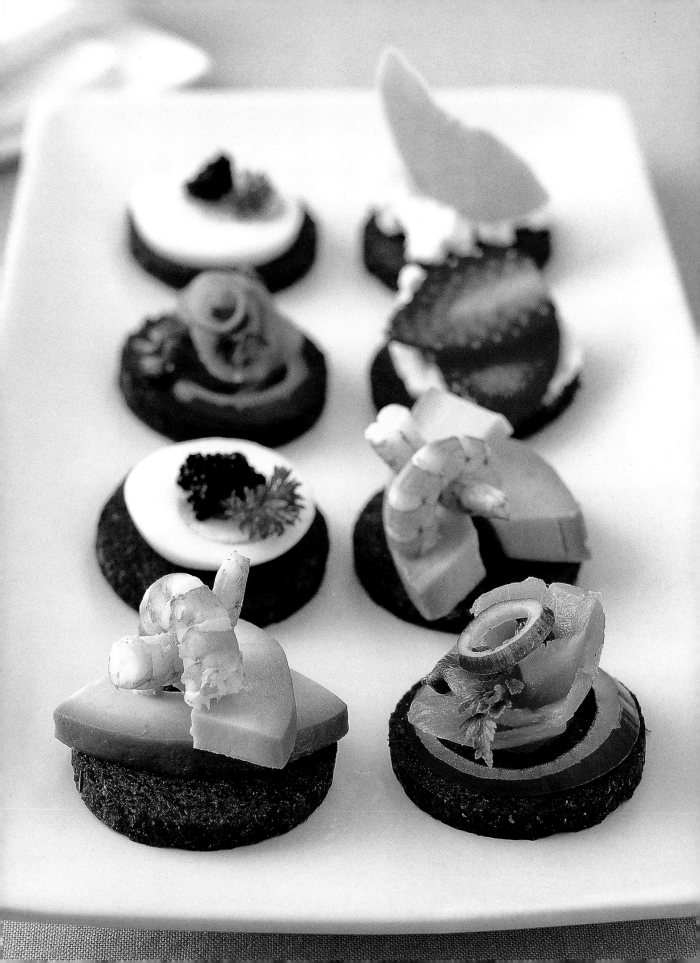

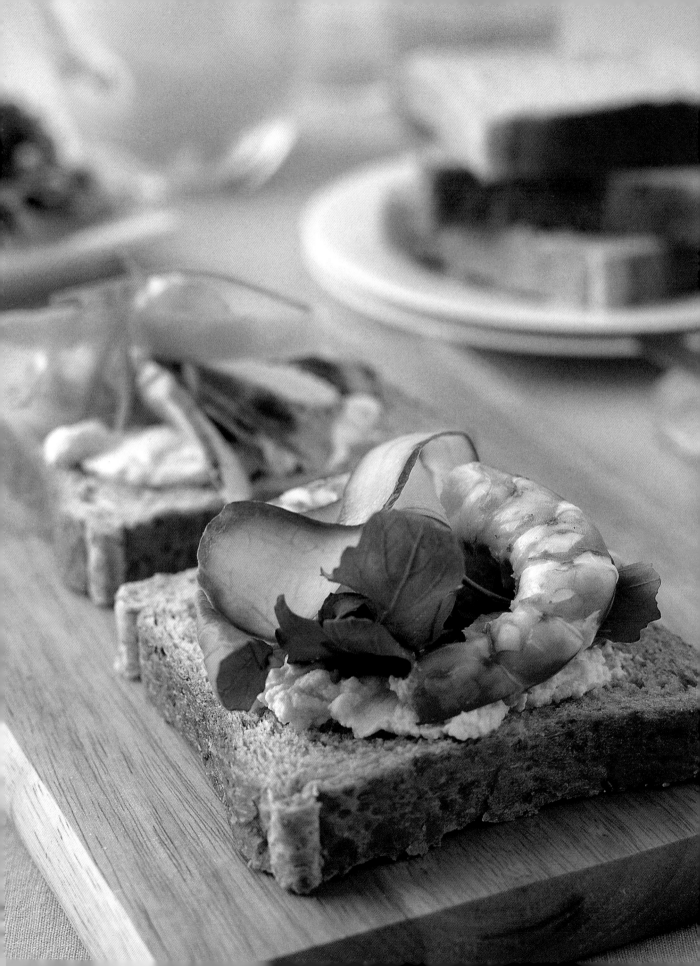

• baby prawns or shrimps and avocado • smoked salmon slices or rolls garnished with capers • sliced hard-boiled egg topped with black caviar and tiny sprigs of parsley • circles or squares of lean ham with asparagus tips • low-fat cottage or ricotta cheese topped with strawberry halves, slices of peach or nectarine, or chopped dried figs or dates.

SANDWICH FILLINGS

Remember when you use any of these delicious fillings, you do not need to use any spread on the bread—and use wholegrain rather than white bread. Use fillings either for closed or open sandwiches.

Cheese
• mixture of grated cheddar cheese, grated apple, carrot, chopped celery and pecans or walnuts mixed with creamy yoghurt dressing (see recipe, page 170) • ricotta cheese with sliced cucumber, tomato and chopped basil • ricotta cheese with chopped celery and walnuts
• mustard, grated cheddar cheese and sliced olives • sliced cheddar cheese, thinly sliced green apple and fresh mango pickle (see recipe, page 172)

Fish
• salmon or tuna in brine, with sliced cucumber or celery, topped with creamy yoghurt dressing (see recipe, page 170) • prawn, ricotta cheese and thinly sliced cucumber • smoked salmon, reduced-fat cream cheese and capers

Meat or chicken
• fresh mango pickle (see recipe, page 172) or mustard topped with thinly sliced cold lean meat
• chopped chicken, chives and parsley bound with creamy yoghurt dressing (see recipe, page 170)
• chopped chicken, walnuts and celery or green capsicum (bell pepper), bound with low-fat natural yoghurt • whole seed mustard, chopped lean ham and grated apple • chopped chicken topped with thinly sliced raw mushrooms and curry dressing (see recipe, page 168)

Egg
• scrambled eggs with finely chopped lean ham • hard-boiled eggs mashed with alfalfa or bean sprouts and curry dressing (see recipe, page 168)

Vegetables
• canned baked beans, lightly mashed and seasoned with tabasco sauce • peanut butter and sliced cucumber or chopped celery • mashed kidney or three-bean mix with chilli, capsicum (bell pepper), cucumber and onion

Sweet fillings
• mashed banana, lemon juice and cinnamon • cottage or ricotta cheese with chopped dried fig

CHICKEN LIVER PÂTÉ

- 250g chicken livers
- ¼ cup (60ml) water
- 1 sprig fresh thyme or
  ¼ teaspoon dried thyme
- 2 bay leaves
- coarsely ground black pepper to
  taste, plus extra to garnish
- salt to taste
- ½ cup (125ml) port

🕐 30 minutes

VARIATION: Replace port with
4 tablespoons each of orange juice
and brandy and add the grated rind
of half an orange.

Chicken liver pâté is usually made with lashings of butter and cream. This recipe avoids additional fats, yet tastes delicious.

METHOD

1. Wash, dry and roughly chop the livers, discarding any greenish portions (which is not a sign of deterioration, but it may discolour the pâté).
2. Bring the water to the boil in a saucepan. Add the livers and stir until sealed, about two minutes.
3. Add the thyme, bay leaves, pepper and salt. Cover, reduce heat and simmer gently for 10 minutes.
4. Add port and simmer, uncovered, for a further three minutes.
5. If using fresh thyme, remove and discard the sprig. Remove and discard bay leaves.
6. Allow mixture to cool slightly. Purée liver and cooking liquids in a food processor or blender.
7. Cover and refrigerate for up to three days.
8. To serve as an appetiser, spoon the pâté into a serving bowl, sprinkle with black pepper, and chill for at least one hour before serving. Surround the dip with sliced fresh vegetables, biscuits or triangles of dry toast.
9. To serve as an entrée, spoon the pâté into small, individual pots or ramekins. Smooth over the surface, sprinkle with black pepper and chill for at least one hour before serving. Place the pots on small plates and arrange a couple of dry toast triangles or crisp biscuits on each plate.

NUTRITION DATA PER SERVING:
77 kcal (324 kJ), CHO 3g, protein 8g, fat 2g.

MOONG DHAL

MAKES 2 CUPS

- 1 cup (190g) dried red lentils
- 3 cups (750ml) water
- ½ teaspoon turmeric
- 1 tomato, peeled and chopped
- 2 teaspoons oil
- ½ teaspoon cumin seeds
- 3 curry leaves (optional)
- 1 onion, finely chopped or minced
- 2 cloves garlic, chopped or finely minced
- 1 tablespoon minced ginger
- 1½ tablespoons curry powder
- salt (optional)
- 1 tablespoon chopped coriander (optional)

⏱ 1 hour

METHOD
1. Wash lentils thoroughly, removing any that float.
2. Put water, lentils, turmeric and chopped tomato in a saucepan, and boil mixture for 20–30 minutes until lentils are soft and the consistency thick. Alternatively, microwave on high for 20 minutes.
3. Heat oil in frying pan, add cumin seeds, curry leaves, onion, garlic and ginger and sauté until golden. Stir in curry powder and sauté for three to four minutes more. If mixture is too thick, add about ½ cup (125ml) boiling water. Combine mixture with the cooked lentils and stir well. Add salt if desired.
4. Just before serving garnish with chopped coriander. Serve hot as a dip with accompaniments (see list, page 59).
5. Cover and refrigerate for up to two days. Reheat before serving.

NUTRITION DATA PER TOTAL:
652 kcal (2728 kJ), CHO 40g, protein 17g, fat 47g.

CHEESE PUFFS

SERVES FOUR

- 2 eggs
- 2 thin slices lean ham, chopped
- 90g reduced-fat cheddar cheese, grated
- 1 small firm tomato, finely chopped
- ½ teaspoon chopped chives
- freshly ground black pepper
- 4 slices of wholegrain bread

⏱ 15 minutes

METHOD
1. Preheat grill.
2. Place eggs in a bowl and beat lightly with a fork.
3. Add remaining ingredients, except bread, and mix.
4. Toast bread on one side, remove from the grill and spread the cheese mixture over the untoasted side of the bread.
5. Grill until the mixture puffs up and browns. Serve hot.

NUTRITION DATA PER SERVING:
187 kcal (784 kJ), CHO 10g, protein 14g, fat 10g.

NACHOS

SERVES FOUR AS AN APPETISER

- 1½ large rounds wholemeal pitta bread
- ¾ cup (100g) grated low-fat mozzarella cheese
- salt and pepper, freshly ground, to taste
- ½ large or 1 small ripe avocado
- 1 tablespoon onion, shallot or spring onion, finely chopped
- 2 tablespoons lemon juice
- 4–5 drops Tabasco sauce
- 2 tablespoons light sour cream
- 2 tablespoons low-fat natural yoghurt
- 3–4 tablespoons commercial tomato-based salsa

⏱ 20–30 minutes

METHOD

1. Split the pitta bread and cut into shapes as for corn chips.
2. Place the pieces of bread on a baking sheet and cook in a low oven until crisp and lightly browned. Alternatively, place a piece of kitchen towel on the microwave turntable. Put six to eight pieces of pitta bread on the towel and microwave on high for 35–45 seconds.
3. Place the dried crisps in a shallow baking dish and sprinkle the cheese over the crisps. Add pepper, and salt if desired.
4. Mash the avocado with the onion, lemon juice, Tabasco sauce, pepper and salt, mixing well so the mixture is fairly smooth. Place in a serving bowl.
5. Combine the light sour cream and yoghurt and spoon into a serving bowl.
6. Spoon the salsa into a serving bowl.
7. Place the crisps in a preheated 180° (350°F) oven until the cheese has melted and the crisps are hot.
8. Serve with the avocado mixture, sour cream mixture and the salsa.

NUTRITION DATA PER SERVING:
335 kcal (1405 kJ), CHO 23g, protein 13.4g, fat 21g.

CHICKEN SPREAD

MAKES 1 CUP

- 1 cup (140g) chopped cooked chicken
- ½ cup (65g) chopped almonds or walnuts
- juice of ½ lemon
- 3 tablespoons low-fat natural yoghurt
- pinch mustard powder
- 1 tablespoon chopped onion
- 1 tablepsoon chopped parsley

⏱ 15 minutes

METHOD

1. Blend all ingredients and refrigerate until ready to serve.
2. Serve on triangles of wholegrain toast, or roll in lettuce to make parcels.
3. Cover and refrigerate any leftover spread for up to two days.

NUTRITION DATA PER TOTAL:
761 kcal (3185 kJ), CHO 8g, protein 68g, fat 51g.

SALMON ROLL

SERVES EIGHT

- 440g can pink salmon
- 125g ricotta cheese
- juice of 1 lemon
- 1 teaspoon curry powder
- ¼ teaspoon salt
- 6 spring onions, chopped
- 1 teaspoon gelatine
- 2 tablespoons hot water
- 1 wholegrain bread stick

⏱ 45 minutes

Eat this on the day you make it because it does not keep.

METHOD

1. Drain liquid from salmon and discard skin and bones.
2. Mash the salmon and mix well with the cheese.
3. Add lemon juice, curry powder, salt and spring onions.
4. Melt gelatine in hot water, cool slightly, and stir into salmon mixture. Chill in refrigerator for 30 minutes.
5. Cut breadstick into two equal lengths, and remove the crusty ends. Hollow out with knife or spoon. Discard the soft centre (or use it to make breadcrumbs).
6. Spoon filling into centres of breadstick and pack in firmly.
7. Wrap in aluminium foil and chill until ready to serve.
8. Slice into 2cm pieces and serve.

NUTRITION DATA PER SERVING:
143 kcal (600 kJ), CHO 6g, protein 15g, fat 7g.

CHINESE PORK DUMPLINGS

MAKES 16 DUMPLINGS

- 200g lean minced pork
- 4 spring onions, finely chopped
- 250g can bamboo shoots, finely chopped
- ½ teaspoon minced fresh ginger
- 1 tablespoon soy sauce
- 1 egg white
- 125g wonton pastry squares
- ¼ cup (60ml) soy sauce mixed with dash of chilli sauce

⏱ 45 minutes

METHOD

1. Combine pork, spring onions, bamboo shoots, ginger, 1 tablespoon soy sauce and egg white.
2. Place a heaped teaspoonful of mixture onto each wonton pastry square; keep unused pastry covered with a damp tea towel while you are working.
3. Squeeze the pastry up around the filling to make a filled-bag shape.
4. Place dumplings in an oiled steamer and cook over boiling water for approximately 20 minutes.
5. Serve with soy and chilli dipping sauce.

NUTRITION DATA PER SERVING:
181 kcal (758 kJ), CHO 23g, protein 17g, fat 2g.

VEGETABLE SAMOSAS

- ◆ 2 medium potatoes, scrubbed and diced
- ◆ 1 medium carrot, scrubbed and diced
- ◆ ½ medium sweet potato, peeled and diced
- ◆ 1 cup (160g) frozen peas
- ◆ 1 medium onion, finely chopped
- ◆ 1 teaspoon olive oil
- ◆ ½ teaspoon turmeric
- ◆ 2 teaspoons curry powder
- ◆ ½ teaspoon coriander
- ◆ ½ teaspoon salt or ½ chicken stock cube
- ◆ 1 teaspoon minced fresh ginger
- ◆ pepper to taste
- ◆ 200g low-fat natural yoghurt
- ◆ 12 sheets filo pastry
- ◆ cucumber, onion and tomato, sliced, for garnish

⏱ 1 hour

Count on serving one to two samosas per person.

METHOD

1. Boil, steam or microwave vegetables, except onion, until tender. Cool.
2. Sauté onion in oil until transparent but not brown. Combine with cooked vegetables in a bowl. Add spices. Check flavour and adjust seasoning to taste.
3. Spread a sheet of filo pastry on the bench and spray lightly with spray oil. Place a second sheet over the first and repeat the procedure. Place a third sheet over this, then cut the pastry in half lengthwise with a sharp knife.
4. Place a generous spoonful of the mixture on one end of the pastry rectangle and fold the filo diagonally to cover the filling. Continue to fold diagonally until all the pastry is folded, making sure that the mixture is totally enclosed.
5. Repeat this procedure until all the pastry is used.
6. Place samosas on a baking sheet and spray lightly with spray oil. Bake in a preheated 180°C (350°F) oven for approximately 15 minutes until brown.
7. Serve with a garnish of sliced cucumber, onion and tomato, or cucumber and yoghurt sauce (see recipe, page 166) or fresh mango pickle (see recipe, page 172).

NUTRITION DATA, PER SERVING (IF FOUR SERVINGS):
252 kcal (1056 kJ), CHO 44g, protein 11g, fat 4g.

SOUPS

Soups can be a nutritious and warming start to a meal, especially on a cold winter's day, the basis of a light meal, or a filling snack between meals or after school. For those who are not keen on vegetables, soups can be a great way to include vegetables in the diet, either as pieces or puréed to a smooth, velvety liquid. Ingredients for soups can be wide-ranging, resulting in thick, hearty meals such as corn chowder (see recipe, page 70), or beef and bean soup (see recipe, page 74), or made into lighter, low calorie meals or snacks like Hungarian cabbage soup (see recipe, page 73). A good stock forms the basis of most soups. This can be made from fresh or frozen vegetables, meat and/or bones. If time is short, however, good pre-prepared stocks are available at most supermarkets.

Some soups need long, slow cooking to develop the flavours, while others are very quick and easy to prepare. Soups lend themselves to preparation ahead of time, and storage in the refrigerator or freezer for later use. Although most of us associate soup with cold winter weather, chilled soups can make a refreshing starter to a summer meal, for example gazpacho (see recipe, page 76).

CHICKEN STOCK

MAKES FOUR CUPS

- 2 medium onions, peeled
- 1 large carrot
- 2 sticks celery
- 1 x 1.5kg boiling fowl
- 8 peppercorns
- 2 bay leaves
- sprig of fresh thyme or
  ¼ teaspoon dried thyme
- 5 sprigs parsley
- 6 cups (1.5litres) water
- salt to taste

⏱ about 3 hours

VARIATION: Just before serving, add
½ cup cooked vermicelli or boiled
rice to the hot soup.

Chicken stock is so useful to have on hand. We use it in many recipes, and it is superior to soup cubes or packet soups. You can also reheat it and serve in cups as a nutritious hot beverage.

METHOD

1. Wash and roughly chop the vegetables.
2. Place all the ingredients in a large saucepan.
3. Over medium heat, slowly bring mixture to the boil. Skim off any scum that rises to the surface. Reduce heat, cover saucepan, and simmer gently for three hours.
4. Strain the soup through a sieve. Reserve meat for another dish. Discard skin, bones and vegetables.
5. Chill in refrigerator overnight and then skim off any congealed fat.

NUTRITION DATA PER SERVING: negligible.

GREEN PEA, SPINACH AND CHICKEN SOUP

SERVES FOUR

- 2 cups (320g) frozen peas
- 3 cups (750ml) chicken stock (see recipe above or use commercial liquid chicken stock)
- 250g packet frozen spinach
- 1 cup (140g) chopped, cooked chicken
- 2 teaspoons curry powder

⏱ 45 minutes

METHOD

1. Cook peas in stock until tender (approximately 15 minutes).
2. Combine in food processor until partly broken down, then return to saucepan.
3. Add spinach and simmer until the spinach is thoroughly heated (approximately 10 minutes).
4. Add chicken and curry powder; bring to the boil and serve.

NUTRITION DATA PER SERVING:
128 kcal (537 kJ), CHO 5g, protein 20g, fat 3g.

MINESTRONE

- 2 medium onions
- 2 medium carrots
- 2 sticks celery
- ½ capsicum (bell pepper)
- 2 medium potatoes
- 1 cup (125g) green beans, sliced
- 1 cup (90g) shredded cabbage
- 4 large tomatoes
- 2 teaspoons olive oil
- 1 cup (250g) dried haricot or cannellini beans
- 4 cups (1 litre) water
- 3 bay leaves
- ½ teaspoon salt
- ¼ teaspoon pepper
- juice of ½ lemon
- 1 teaspoon dried mixed herbs or 2 teaspoons fresh mixed herbs

⏱ 2 hours

There are dozens of versions of this soup. This one has all the key ingredients of the classic version. To make this soup into a meal-in-one, you can add 2 cups (400g) cooked macaroni just before serving. This provides additional long-acting carbohydrate.

METHOD

1. Peel and chop vegetables.
2. Heat oil in saucepan.
3. Add onions and cook until lightly browned.
4. Add carrots, celery capsicum (bell pepper) and potatoes. Cook until lightly coloured.
5. Add green beans, cabbage and tomatoes. Cook until just tender.
6. Add dried beans, water, herbs and lemon juice.
7. Simmer with lid on until beans are tender (approximately 1 hour).
8. Check for flavour and adjust seasoning to taste.
9. Serve with wholemeal breadstick.

NUTRITION DATA PER SERVING:
264 kcal (1105 kJ), CHO 40g, protein 17g, fat 4g.

CORN CHOWDER

SERVES FOUR

- ◆ 2 teaspoons margarine
- ◆ 1 large onion, peeled and chopped
- ◆ 2 medium potatoes, peeled and cut into 1cm dice
- ◆ 1 chicken stock cube
- ◆ pinch mixed dried herbs or ½ teaspoon chopped fresh mixed herbs
- ◆ pepper to taste
- ◆ 440g can corn kernels
- ◆ ½ cup (125ml) water
- ◆ 1½ (375ml) cups skimmed or semi-skimmed milk
- ◆ 4 teaspoons cornflour (cornstarch)

⏱ 45 minutes

METHOD

1. Melt margarine in saucepan. Add onion and cook over low heat until translucent.
2. Add potatoes, stock cube, herbs, pepper, the corn and its liquid and the water to the saucepan.
3. Cover and simmer until potatoes are tender (approximately 15 minutes). Add milk.
4. In a small bowl, blend cornflour with a little water to a smooth paste. Add to the soup.
5. Bring to the boil, then simmer until slightly thickened, stirring from time to time.
6. Sprinkle with parsley and serve.

NUTRITION DATA PER SERVING:
246 kcal (1032 kJ), CHO 44g, protein 8g, fat 4g.

CHINESE CHICKEN AND SWEETCORN SOUP

SERVES FOUR

- ◆ 2 teaspoons oil
- ◆ 2 skinless chicken fillets, finely sliced
- ◆ 2 cloves garlic, crushed
- ◆ 1 teaspoon chopped ginger
- ◆ 4 cups (1 litre) chicken stock (see recipe page 68 or use commercial liquid stock)
- ◆ 425g can creamed sweetcorn
- ◆ 1 egg, lightly beaten
- ◆ 3 spring onions, for garnish

⏱ 45 minutes

METHOD

1. Place oil in saucepan and heat until moderately hot.
2. Lightly brown sliced chicken, garlic and ginger. Don't overcook.
3. Add stock and bring to boil.
4. Add creamed corn and simmer for 10 minutes.
5. Remove from heat when ready to serve, then quickly stir in egg to make long strands.
6. Garnish with chopped spring onions.

NUTRITION DATA PER SERVING:
246 kcal (1029 kJ), CHO 26g, protein 17g, fat 8g.

HOT AND SOUR SOUP

SERVES FOUR

- 3 chicken fillets
- 2½ tablespoons white vinegar
- 2 teaspoons oil
- 125g firm tofu (soybean curd),
  cut into small cubes
- 4 cups (1 litre) chicken stock (see
  recipe page 68 or use commercial
  liquid stock)
- ½ medium red capsicum
  (bell pepper), sliced
- 125g button mushrooms
- 125g can bamboo shoots, drained
- 4 spring onions, chopped
- 2 tablespoons cornflour (cornstarch)
- 1 egg
- soy sauce, to serve

⏱ 30 minutes

METHOD

1. With a sharp knife, slice chicken very finely and place in
   a bowl with the vinegar.
2. Place oil in heavy saucepan over a high heat. Add tofu
   and stir-fry until tender (about three minutes). Remove
   from saucepan.
3. Pour chicken stock into saucepan with capsicum,
   mushrooms, bamboo shoots and spring onions. Heat to
   boiling, cover and simmer 10 minutes or until vegetables
   are tender.
4. Add chicken and tofu, heat to boiling.
5. Mix cornflour and a small amount of water and slowly stir
   cornflour mixture into boiling soup.
6. Cook, stirring constantly, until slightly thickened. Remove
   from heat.
7. Beat egg in a small bowl then slowly pour egg mixture
   into soup, stirring quickly until egg swirls and has just set.
8. Spoon soup into individual bowls and add a dash of
   soy sauce.

NUTRITION DATA PER SERVING:
317 kcal (1328 kJ), CHO 8g, protein 28g, fat 19g.

SINGAPORE NOODLE SOUP

SERVES FOUR

- 300g green prawns
- 3 cups (750ml) water
- 2 cups (500ml) chicken stock (see recipe page 68 or use commercial liquid stock)
- 2 teaspoons sesame oil
- 2 cloves garlic, finely chopped
- ½ teaspoon finely chopped fresh ginger
- 100g fine egg noodles
- 180g lean barbecued pork, cut into thin strips
- 1 cup (90g) bean sprouts, washed and drained
- 12 spinach leaves, washed and drained
- ½ teaspoon five spice powder
- 110g can crab meat
- 4 spring onions, finely chopped
- ½ cup finely diced cucumber

⏱ 45 minutes

Although a soup, this dish makes an ideal light meal.

METHOD

1. Shell and de-vein prawns. Wash shells and heads well and shake dry.
2. Bring water to boil, add shells and heads, cover and boil for 20 minutes. Strain.
3. Combine prawn and chicken stocks.
4. Heat oil and gently fry garlic and ginger until starting to brown.
5. Add stock and prawns and simmer for three minutes.
6. Add noodles and simmer for a further five minutes.
7. Add pork, bean sprouts, spinach and five spice powder and simmer for two minutes.
8. Pour into a large bowl and garnish with crab meat, spring onions and cucumber.

NUTRITION DATA PER SERVING:
334 kcal (1397 kJ), CHO 19g, protein 34g, fat 13g.

HUNGARIAN CABBAGE SOUP

SERVES FOUR

- ◆ 3 cups (750ml) chicken stock (see recipe page 68 or use commercial liquid stock)
- ◆ 1 cup (90g) finely shredded red cabbage or ¾ cup (115g) canned red cabbage, drained
- ◆ 3 small onions, thinly sliced
- ◆ 1 clove garlic, crushed
- ◆ 2 large tomatoes, peeled and quartered
- ◆ 1 large apple, peeled and chopped
- ◆ coarsely ground black pepper, to taste
- ◆ ¼ teaspoon ground allspice
- ◆ chives, chopped, to garnish

⏱ 45 minutes

This is a simple, filling and aromatic soup with just a hint of sweetness, ideal for cold winter nights. Eaten with wholegrain bread, it makes a warming supper.

METHOD

1. Place stock in a large saucepan and bring to the boil.
2. Add all other ingredients. Cover and simmer for 30 minutes.
3. Serve, garnished with a sprinkling of chopped chives.

NUTRITION DATA PER SERVING:
51 kcal (213 kJ), CHO 10g, protein 2g, fat trace.

BROCCOLI AND SWEETCORN SOUP

SERVES FOUR

- ◆ 1 large head broccoli
- ◆ 2 cups (500ml) chicken stock (see recipe page 68 or use commercial liquid stock) or vegetable stock
- ◆ 440g can creamed sweetcorn
- ◆ 1 stick celery, finely chopped
- ◆ 6 spring onions, finely sliced
- ◆ ½ teaspoon salt (optional)
- ◆ pepper to taste
- ◆ chives, chopped, to garnish

Note the high proportion of complex carbohydrate in this delicious soup. Use the chicken stock recipe on page 68 for a superior result.

METHOD

1. Break the broccoli into florets and cook it in stock until tender (approximately 10 minutes).
2. Blend until smooth in food processor.
3. Add creamed sweetcorn, celery, spring onions and seasonings.
4. Reheat and serve, garnished with chopped chives.

NUTRITION DATA PER SERVING:
182 kcal (760 kJ), CHO 30g, protein 9g, fat 3g.

PORK AND VEGETABLE NOODLE SOUP

SERVES FOUR

- ◆ 200g bacon bones
- ◆ 4 cups (1 litre) water
- ◆ 250g pork fillet, diced
- ◆ 1 medium carrot, grated
- ◆ 2 sticks celery, chopped
- ◆ ½ parsnip, grated
- ◆ ½ turnip, grated
- ◆ 1 medium leek, chopped
- ◆ 2 tablespoons chopped parsley
- ◆ ½ teaspoon black pepper
- ◆ 85g packet instant noodles
- ◆ spring onions, chopped, to garnish

🕐 2 hours

METHOD

1. Place bacon bones and water in saucepan and bring to boil. Simmer for one hour. Strain stock and discard the bones.
2. Chill stock to set any fat, and remove.
3. Heat saucepan and dry fry pork fillet until browned.
4. Add pork, carrot, celery, parsnip, turnip, leek, parsley and black pepper to stock.
5. Cook until meat and vegetables are tender.
6. Add noodles and cook a further five to ten minutes or until noodles are tender.
7. Spoon into individual bowls and garnish with chopped spring onions.

NUTRITION DATA PER SERVING:
151 kcal (633 kJ), CHO 16g, protein 18g, fat 2g.

BEEF AND BEAN SOUP

SERVES FOUR

- ◆ 250g lean minced beef
- ◆ 1 medium onion, diced
- ◆ 1 small clove garlic
- ◆ 2 sticks celery, diced
- ◆ 410g can tomatoes
- ◆ 1 tablespoon tomato puree
- ◆ 3 cups (750ml) water
- ◆ ½ teaspoon dried oregano, or
  1 teaspoon fresh oregano
- ◆ ½ teaspoon paprika
- ◆ ½ teaspoon ground cumin
- ◆ 2 teaspoons white vinegar
- ◆ 440g can kidney beans, drained

🕐 1 hour

METHOD

1. Dry fry meat. Add onion and garlic and cook until juices evaporate and beef is well browned.
2. Add celery, tomatoes, tomato puree, water, oregano, paprika, cumin and vinegar.
3. Bring to boil. Add beans and reduce heat to low, cover and simmer 30 minutes.

NUTRITION DATA PER SERVING:
202 kcal (844 kJ), CHO 17g, protein 26g, fat 3g.

SOUPER DOUPER PUMPKIN SOUP

SERVES FOUR

- 750g pumpkin, peeled and cut into pieces
- 1 large leek, sliced
- 3 cups (750ml) chicken stock
- 2 teaspoons mixed dried herbs or 3 teaspoons fresh herbs
- ½ teaspoon coarsley ground black pepper
- ½ teaspoon ground nutmeg
- ½ teaspoon coriander
- ½ teaspoon salt
- 2 tablespoons lemon juice
- 2 tablespoons chopped parsley

⏱ 1 hour

METHOD

1. Place all ingredients except lemon juice and parsley in a saucepan.
2. Bring to the boil and simmer until pumpkin is tender (approximately 20 minutes).
3. Cool slightly, blend in food processor or blender until smooth.
4. Add lemon juice and parsley. Check taste, add salt if needed.
5. Serve with herby corn muffins (see recipe page 198).

NUTRITION DATA PER SERVING:
82 kcal (342 kJ), CHO 14g, protein 5g, fat 1g.

ORANGE BORSCHT

SERVES FOUR

- 3 cups (450g) peeled and grated beetroot
- 3 cups (750ml) chicken stock
- 1 cup (250ml) unsweetened orange juice
- 1 cup (250ml) unsweetened tomato juice
- 1 sprig fresh thyme or ½ teaspoon dried thyme
- ground black pepper
- 2 tablespoons chopped parsley, to garnish

⏱ 30 minutes

Beetroot soup (borscht) is East European in origin and would, traditionally, have been eaten with plain boiled potatoes on the side. You can also add a spoonful of low-fat natural yoghurt to each bowl just before you serve the soup.

METHOD

1. Place beetroot and stock in saucepan and bring to the boil. Simmer for 20 minutes.
2. Strain stock into a clean saucepan and add 1 cup of the cooked beetroot. Discard the remaining beetroot.
3. Add the juices, thyme and pepper.
4. Bring to boil and remove sprig of thyme.
5. Serve in bowls and sprinkle with chopped parsley.

NUTRITION DATA PER SERVING:
63 kcal (263 kJ), CHO 13g, protein 2g, fat trace.

GAZPACHO

SERVES FOUR

This tangy soup can also be served hot with toasted croutons.

- 1 small cucumber, peeled
- 3 spring onions
- ½ red capsicum (bell pepper)
- ½ green capsicum (bell pepper)
- 2 sticks of celery
- 4 medium ripe tomatoes, or one 425g can of tomatoes
- 1 medium white onion
- 1 cup (250ml) tomato juice
- 1 tablespoon ground black pepper
- 1–2 teaspoons Tabasco sauce, according to taste
- chopped parsley, for garnish

⏱ 25 minutes

METHOD

1. Finely chop half the cucumber, spring onions, one quarter of each capsicum, one stick of celery and one tomato. Set aside.
2. Roughly chop all remaining vegetables and place in food processor with tomato juice, pepper and Tabasco sauce and blend until smooth.
3. Add finely chopped vegetables, mix and chill well.
4. Serve chilled, garnished with chopped parsley.

NUTRITION DATA PER SERVING:
47 kcal (195 kJ), CHO 8g, protein 3g, fat trace.

MOROCCAN LENTIL SOUP

SERVES FOUR TO SIX

- 1 cup (190g) red lentils
- 1 tablespoon olive oil
- 1 Spanish (red) onion, finely chopped
- 2 cloves garlic, crushed
- 1 teaspoon ground coriander
- 1 teaspoon ground cumin
- 1 large carrot, grated
- 1 tomato, finely chopped
- 1 potato, cut into small dice
- 4 cups (1 litre) vegetable or meat stock
- 2 tablespoons lemon juice
- freshly ground black pepper
- salt to taste
- 3–4 tablespoons chopped coriander

⏱ 1 hour 20 minutes

METHOD

1. Rinse the lentils and set aside.
2. Add the oil to a large saucepan and heat.
3. Add the onion, garlic and ground spices and cook, stirring, until the onion is clear.
4. Add the carrot, tomato, potato, lentils and stock. Bring to the boil, then reduce the heat and simmer until the vegetables are tender and the lentils soft.
5. Add the lemon juice, check the flavour and add ground black pepper and salt to taste.
6. Stir in the fresh coriander and serve.

NUTRITION DATA PER SERVING:
146 kcal (613 kJ), CHO 17g, protein 9g, fat 4g.

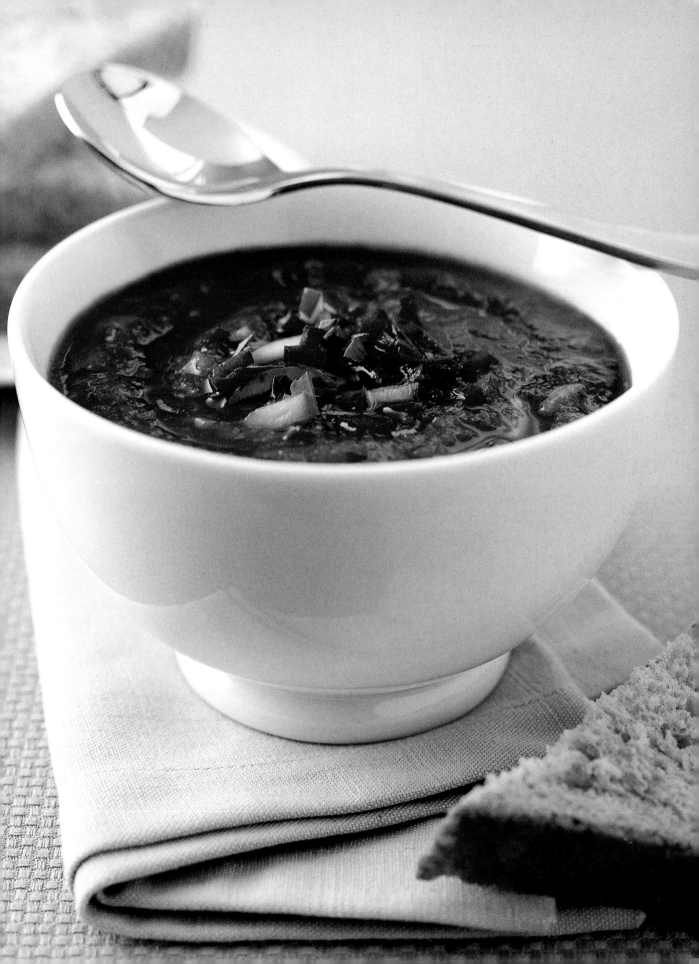

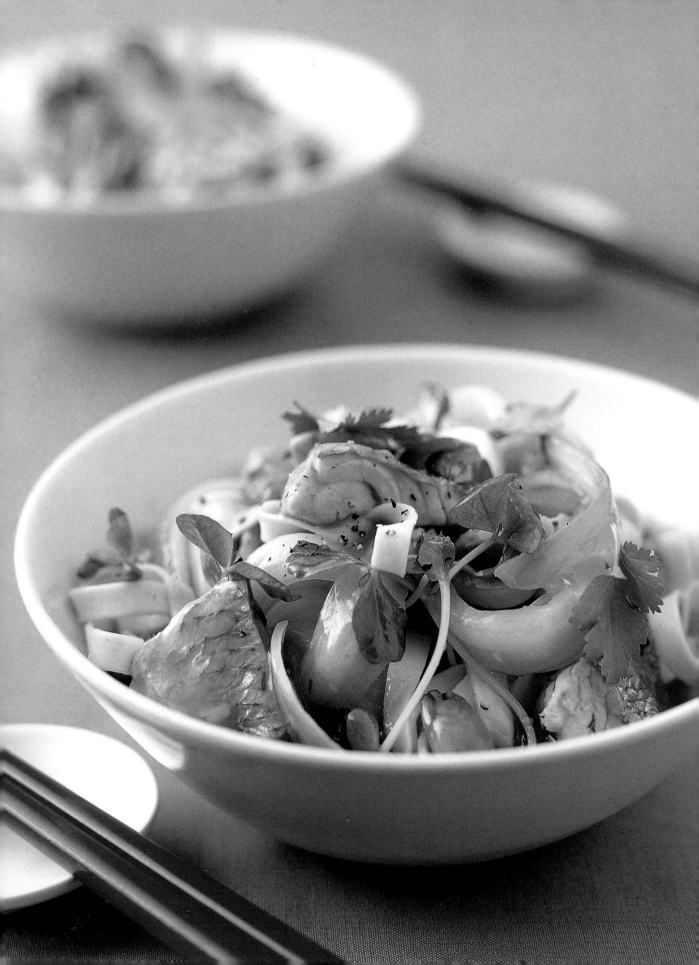

FISH AND SEAFOOD

Fish and seafood contain plenty of protein, vitamins and minerals and little fat. This gives them a calorie/energy value less than an equivalent serving of meat and makes fish and seafood an invaluable, and delicious, part of your regular meal plan. Fish is also a valuable addition to meals because of its heart-healthy properties. There are various methods of cooking both fish and seafood:

Baking

Place the fish (whole, cutlets or fillets) in a shallow casserole and flavour it to taste, for instance with a sliced onion, a bay leaf, herbs of your choice, a few peppercorns and a little salt (optional). Then pour over approximately 125ml–250ml liquid depending on the amount of fish. The liquid can be semi-skimmed milk, wine or tomato juice. Bake, covered, at 180°C (350°F) for 15–20 minutes or until the fish flakes when you test it with a fork. Alternatively, place the fish on foil, sprinkle with lemon juice and herbs, seal, and then cook as above without any additional liquid.

Grilling

Allow five to eight minutes for fillets, cutlets, kebabs or small fish; 10 minutes for medium-sized whole fish and 15–20 minutes for large whole fish. Turn the fish once or twice while it cooks, ensuring it doesn't overcook. Grilled fish is delicious cooked with no more than a sprinkling of herbs, lemon juice, black pepper and a little salt (optional), or use one of the marinade recipes on p.161.

Poaching

Place the fish in a shallow saucepan with a lid, add just enough liquid (milk, stock or wine or a combination of any two of these) to barely cover the fish and then season it to taste. For instance, add sliced onion, bay leaf, peppercorns, ground black pepper, parsley and a sliced carrot for a wonderfully flavoursome result. Cover and simmer gently on the stove for five to eight minutes for thin fillets, or about 10 minutes for thicker fillets. Remove from the heat immediately and use the poaching liquid as the base for a sauce.

Microwaving

Cover fish with 60ml liquid such as wine, stock or semi-skimmed milk, flavour as for poaching, cover with plastic wrap and cook on high. Allow three minutes for small fillets, five to seven minutes for larger fillets or small whole fish and 10–12 minutes for large whole fish. Arrange seafood in a single layer in a shallow dish. Cover with plastic wrap and cook on medium until opaque (approximately three to four minutes). Stand, covered, for five minutes before serving.

Fish with Various Sauces

Grill four fillets of white fish such as snapper, flathead, whiting or sea perch on both sides until cooked (approximately eight to ten minutes). Alternatively, cover and microwave on medium-high for four to six minutes. Serve with a sauce such as green champagne (see recipe, page 168), black bean (see recipe, page 165), ratatouille (see recipe, page 165) or sweet and sour (see recipe, page 167).

STIR-FRIED BOK CHOY WITH FISH AND ALMONDS

SERVES FOUR

- ◆ 4 fillets white fish (e.g snapper or flathead), cut into bite-sized pieces
- ◆ 2 teaspoons finely chopped fresh ginger or paste
- ◆ 2 tablespoons chopped fresh coriander
- ◆ juice and grated rind of 1 lemon
- ◆ 3 tablespoons teriyaki sauce
- ◆ 1 cup (250ml) fish stock or water
- ◆ 1 bunch baby bok choy, roughly chopped
- ◆ 1 medium Spanish (red) onion, peeled and cut into wedges
- ◆ 1 cup (60g) snowpea shoots or bean sprouts
- ◆ 1 tablespoon cornflour (cornstarch)
- ◆ 2 tablespoons water
- ◆ black pepper
- ◆ 200g pasta (e.g. conchiglie or tagliatelle), cooked
- ◆ 75g toasted almonds, for garnish
- ◆ 4 sprigs coriander, for garnish

🕐 30 minutes

VARIATION: Replace all or part of fish with scallops, chicken, or tofu.

METHOD

1. Marinate fish in ginger, coriander, lemon juice, rind and teriyaki sauce for 15 minutes.
2. Heat stock in wok, add fish and marinade and bring to boil.
3. Reduce to simmer, add bok choy and onion and stir-fry for about two minutes or until vegetables are just tender.
4. Add snow pea shoots or bean sprouts and continue to stir-fry until all ingredients are warmed through.
5. Mix cornflour and water to form paste and add.
6. Stir until sauce cooks and thickens.
7. Season with black pepper to taste.
8. Add cooked pasta. Stir-fry to mix ingredients evenly until warmed through.
9. Serve on warmed plates and garnish with almonds and sprigs of coriander.

NUTRITION DATA PER SERVING:
274 kcal (1148 kJ), CHO 18g, protein 12g, fat 22g.

PIQUANT FISH IN FOIL

SERVES FOUR

- ◆ 4 large fillets of fish (e.g. haddock or cod), or small whole fish (e.g. whiting or bream)
- ◆ 2 teaspoons finely chopped fresh tarragon (or ½ teaspoon dried tarragon)
- ◆ 1 tablespoon very finely chopped parsley
- ◆ coarsely ground black pepper, to taste
- ◆ 1 medium onion, thinly sliced
- ◆ 1 lemon, thinly sliced
- ◆ juice of 1 lemon
- ◆ 2 tablespoons dry white wine

⏱ 30–40 minutes

This is a wonderful way to prepare fresh fish. Serve it with jacket potatoes and a crisp salad.

METHOD

1. Lightly grease, or spray with non-stick cooking spray, four pieces of foil large enough to completely wrap the fish fillets.
2. Place the fish fillets on the pieces of foil. Sprinkle each fillet with the herbs and black pepper. Arrange several onion rings on top of each fillet and top with one or two slices of lemon.
3. Mix lemon juice and white wine and pour over the fish.
4. Wrap each fillet in foil, sealing along the top, so that the juices aren't lost during cooking or when opening the foil.
5. Place the foil parcels, sealed side up, on a baking tray. Bake in a preheated 180°C (350°F) oven or barbecue over glowing coals for 30 minutes.
6. Open foil along the sealing edge and serve immediately.

NUTRITION DATA PER SERVING:
149 kcal (623 kJ), CHO 2g, protein 27g, fat 3g.

CAJUN FISH

SERVES FOUR

- ◆ 4 pieces firm-fleshed fish
- ◆ cajun spice mixture
- ◆ spray oil

⏱ 15 minutes

METHOD

1. Heat a barbecue plate or griller until really hot—it should be smoking hot.
2. Skin the fish if necessary, then coat each piece of fish well with the spice mixture.
3. Spray the hot plate with oil, then place the fish on the hot surface.
4. Cook the fish on one side for two to three minutes, depending on the thickness of the fish, then turn over and cook on the other side for one to two minutes, or until just cooked. The surface of the fish will be black.
5. Serve the fish on a platter of wild rice pilaf (see recipe, page 139), accompanied by lemon or lime wedges.

NUTRITION DATA PER SERVING:
81 kcal (338 kJ), CHO 0g, protein 16g, fat 2g.

SEAFOOD PASTA

SERVES FOUR

- ◆ 300g pasta (e.g. spaghetti, tagliatelle or macaroni)
- ◆ 2 tablespoons water
- ◆ ½ medium onion, chopped
- ◆ 1 clove garlic, crushed
- ◆ 1 cup (250ml) skimmed milk
- ◆ 2 teaspoons cornflour (cornstarch)
- ◆ 1½ cups (230g) mixed cooked seafood (oysters, calamari, shrimps, clams, scallops)
- ◆ 1 tablespoon chopped parsley
- ◆ coarsely ground black pepper
- ◆ salt to taste

⏱ 30 minutes

METHOD

1. Fill a large saucepan two-thirds full with water, and bring to a rapid boil. Add pasta, and boil rapidly for 10–12 minutes until al dente (tender, but still firm to bite).
2. While the pasta is cooking, prepare the sauce. In a medium saucepan, boil the 2 tablespoons of water. Add the onion and garlic and cook until tender.
3. In a small bowl, blend 1 tablespoon of the milk with the cornflour to make a smooth paste. Then stir in the remainder of the milk. Add mixture to the onion and garlic, and stir constantly over medium heat until sauce thickens.
4. Over medium heat, add all the remaining ingredients, and stir to combine and heat through.
5. Drain the pasta and add to the sauce. Toss gently to combine.
6. Serve at once.

NUTRITION DATA PER SERVING:
357 kcal (1495 kJ), CHO 48g, protein 31g, fat 4g.

PASTA AND SMOKED TROUT

SERVES FOUR

- ◆ 250g fettucine pasta
- ◆ 1 medium smoked trout
- ◆ ½ cup (125ml) dry white wine
- ◆ ½ teaspoon granulated garlic (or 1 clove of garlic, chopped)
- ◆ ½ teaspoon dry mustard
- ◆ ½ quantity white sauce (see recipe, page 162)
- ◆ 1 tablespoon chopped capers, parsley, chives or spring onions, for garnish

⏱ 30–35 minutes

METHOD

1. Boil fettucine in water as directed on the pack, and drain.
2. While pasta is cooking, skin the trout and remove the flesh from the bones by lifting it off with a fork. Break the flesh into bite size pieces.
3. Mix wine, garlic and mustard, and bring to the boil in large saucepan. Add the white sauce and gently reheat.
4. Add the fettucine and mix through, reheating gently.
5. Add the fish, mixing carefully. Turn onto a serving dish and sprinkle with your choice of garnish.

NUTRITION DATA PER SERVING:
356 kcal (1490 kJ), CHO 48 g, protein 28g, fat 5g.

STUFFED TROUT

SERVES FOUR

- ◆ 4 small trout, ready to cook
- ◆ juice of 2 lemons
- ◆ 1 cup (60g) soft wholegrain breadcrumbs
- ◆ 2 tablespoons chopped mixed fresh herbs (e.g. thyme, parsley, marjoram)
- ◆ 4 spring onions, finely chopped
- ◆ 1 tablespoon finely chopped celery
- ◆ 2 tablespoons finely chopped green capsicum (bell pepper)
- ◆ 4 mushrooms, finely chopped
- ◆ 1 teaspoon ground black pepper

⏱ 20 minutes

Serve the trout with plenty of pasta, rice or potatoes, plus a salad, for a memorable meal.

METHOD
1. Wash fish.
2. Place each fish on a piece of aluminium foil large enough to wrap it up completely.
3. Pour lemon juice over the outside and inside of fish.
4. Combine all other ingredients in a mixing bowl.
5. Divide mixture into four and pack a quarter of the mixture into the cavity of each fish.
6. Wrap firmly in foil. Seal edges carefully. Alternatively, if you prefer to use the microwave, use a large shallow microwave dish instead of the foil and secure the cavity of each fish with toothpicks. Cover dish with plastic film.
7. Bake in a preheated 180°C (350°F) oven or under the grill until cooked through (approximately 10–15 minutes). If using the microwave, cook on medium-high for 8–12 minutes and stand, covered, for five minutes before serving.

NUTRITION DATA PER SERVING:
122 kcal (511 kJ), CHO 1g, protein 23g, fat 3g.

FISH IN ORANGE SAUCE

SERVES FOUR

- ◆ juice of 2 oranges
- ◆ juice of 1 lemon
- ◆ 1 teaspoon margarine
- ◆ ¼ teaspoon black pepper, coarsely ground
- ◆ 4 fillets fish
- ◆ small quantity of plain flour

⏱ 15 minutes

METHOD
1. Place juices, margarine and pepper in pan.
2. Cook until slightly reduced.
3. Dust fish with flour.
4. Add to sauce and poach until just cooked, turning once.
5. Lift out onto serving plates. Spoon sauce over the fish.

NUTRITION DATA PER SERVING:
166 kcal (693 kJ), CHO 4g, protein 27g, fat 4g.

WHOLE FISH IN GINGER

SERVES FOUR

- ◆ 1kg whole fish (e.g. snapper or trout), gutted and scaled, but with head intact
- ◆ 2 teaspoons chopped fresh ginger
- ◆ 1 clove garlic, crushed
- ◆ ¼ cup (60ml) soy sauce
- ◆ juice of 1 lemon
- ◆ ¾ cup (190ml) dry white wine
- ◆ 4 spring onions, sliced lengthways lemon slices, for garnish

⏱ 40 minutes

METHOD

1. Using a very sharp knife, score the skin of the fish on each side, three or four times, at equal intervals and at an angle to the backbone.
2. Place fish on its side in a flat dish, or support it upright with wooden skewers.
3. Combine remaining ingredients to make a marinade, and pour over the fish.
4. Bake the fish, uncovered, in a 180°C (350°F) oven for 30 minutes or until fish flakes when tested with a fork. Baste frequently with the marinade during cooking. Alternatively, cover with plastic film and microwave on high for 15 minutes.
5. Serve the fish whole with cooking juices and garnished with lemon slices. Accompany with boiled brown rice and a green salad.

NUTRITION DATA PER SERVING:
119 kcal (497 kJ), CHO 1g, protein 22g, fat 3g.

MUSSELS À LA GRECQUE

SERVES FOUR

- ◆ 2 teaspoons olive oil
- ◆ 2 medium leeks, sliced
- ◆ 3 large peeled tomatoes or 425g can tomatoes, chopped
- ◆ 1 tablespoon tomato paste
- ◆ ¼ teaspoon ground basil
- ◆ ½ teaspoon ground oregano
- ◆ ground black pepper to taste
- ◆ salt to taste (not needed if you use canned tomatoes)
- ◆ 1½ kg mussels in shells, scrubbed and beards removed

⏱ 15–20 minutes

Black mussels are ideal for this recipe. However, it is also excellent with clams or pipis. Green-lipped mussels are also perfect for cooking this way.

METHOD

1. Heat oil in a saucepan and sauté leeks until tender.
2. Add tomatoes, tomato paste, basil, oregano, pepper and salt (if desired).
3. Bring to the boil and add mussels.
4. Cover and cook until shells open (this takes only a few minutes).
5. Serve in bowls with crusty bread.

NUTRITION DATA PER SERVING:
173 kcal (723 kJ), CHO 6g, protein 25g, fat 5g.

PAELLA

SERVES EIGHT

- ◆ 2 teaspoons olive oil
- ◆ 8 small skinless chicken pieces (no wings)
- ◆ pinch salt and black pepper
- ◆ 1 large onion, chopped
- ◆ 2 large tomatoes, chopped
- ◆ 1 teaspoon chopped, crushed or minced garlic
- ◆ ¼ teaspoon saffron powder or a pinch of saffron threads
- ◆ 2 cups (410g) basmati rice
- ◆ 2 cups (500ml) water
- ◆ 1 chicken stock cube
- ◆ 1 small green or red capsicum (bell pepper), cut into strips
- ◆ 1 cup (160g) frozen peas
- ◆ 12 cooked king prawns, heads removed, shelled and cleaned (tails left on)

⏱ 2–3 hours

This is a wonderful dinner party or luncheon dish served with a green salad and crusty wholemeal bread.

METHOD

1. Heat oil in frying pan.
2. Sprinkle chicken pieces lightly with black pepper and a pinch of salt (if desired).
3. Add to frying pan and brown well on all sides. Remove from the frying pan and set aside on a plate.
4. Add onion to pan and brown.
5. Add tomato and garlic and cook until soft.
6. Add saffron and rice. Stir.
7. Pour in water and stock cube, and mix well.
8. Spoon into a large shallow casserole dish.
9. Stir capsicum strips, peas and chicken pieces into mixture.
10. Cover and cook in a preheated 200°C (400°F) oven until rice is cooked through and liquid absorbed (approximately 1–2 hours).
11. Just before serving, add the prawns and allow to heat through. Serve immediately from the casserole dish.

NUTRITION DATA PER SERVING:
313 kcal (1312 kJ), CHO 41g, protein 24g, fat 5g.

SALMON MORNAY

SERVES FOUR

- ◆ 440g can salmon
- ◆ 4 spring onions, chopped
- ◆ 4 tablespoons lemon juice
- ◆ 2 stalks celery, finely chopped
- ◆ 2 tablespoons freshly grated
  parmesan cheese
- ◆ 1 quantity cheese sauce (see
  recipe, page 163)
- ◆ 2 hard-boiled eggs, chopped,
  for garnish

⏱ 45 minutes

METHOD

1. Mix salmon, spring onions, lemon juice and celery in a shallow casserole or mornay dish.
2. Add parmesan cheese to sauce and pour over salmon mixture. Mix well.
3. Bake in a preheated 180°C (350°F) oven for 30 minutes. Alternatively, cover and microwave on medium for 12–14 minutes, and stand, covered, for five minutes before serving.
4. Sprinkle with chopped eggs and serve.

NUTRITION DATA PER SERVING:
291 kcal (1219 kJ), CHO 12g, protein 32g, fat 13g.

CRAB AND COURGETTE QUICHE

SERVES FOUR

- ◆ 1 quantity wholemeal pastry (see
  recipe, page 200)
- ◆ 170g can crab meat
- ◆ 1 courgette, sliced
- ◆ 2 spring onions, chopped
- ◆ ¼ cup ricotta cheese
- ◆ 4 eggs
- ◆ 1 cup (250ml) skimmed milk
- ◆ 1 cup (250ml) low-fat natural yoghurt
- ◆ pepper to taste
- ◆ ¼ teaspoon salt (optional)

⏱ 45–60 minutes

VARIATION: You can make this quiche just as successfully with shrimps in place of the crab, or using fresh seafood instead of canned. Asparagus or mushrooms make a delicious substitute for the courgette.

METHOD

1. Roll out pastry and line a 25cm flan dish.
2. Place crab meat, sliced courgette and spring onions over base of pastry.
3. Blend all other ingredients and pour over filling.
4. Bake in a preheated 180°C (350°F) oven for 30–45 minutes or until filling is set.

NUTRITION DATA PER SERVING:
654 kcal (2737 kJ), CHO 56g, protein 30g, fat 34g.

SEAFOOD STIR-FRY

SERVES FOUR

- 500g mixed seafood
- 2 red chillis, de-seeded and finely chopped, or 1 teaspoon minced chilli
- 1 teaspoon finely chopped or minced fresh ginger
- 1 tablespoon sweet sherry
- 1 tablespoon soy sauce
- 200g thin spaghetti or noodles
- 1 onion, peeled and sliced
- ½ cup (45g) sliced Chinese or green cabbage
- ½ cup (60g) snow peas or green beans, topped and tailed
- ½ red capsicum, seeded and sliced
- ½ cup (35g) thinly sliced mushrooms
- ½ cup (125ml) fish stock or water
- ½ cup (45g) bean sprouts
- 2 teaspoons oil
- 2 teaspoons cornflour
- 2 tablespoons water
- salt and ground black pepper to taste

⏱ 25 minutes

VARIATION: Replace all or part of the mixed seafood with thin strips of pork or chicken, green prawns or tofu. A few almonds or cashew nuts could be added for variety of taste and texture.

METHOD

1. Combine seafood with chilli, ginger, sherry and soy sauce and marinate for ten minutes. Drain juices and reserve.
2. Cook spaghetti or noodles until tender, drain, rinse and keep warm.
3. While pasta is cooking, combine all vegetables except bean sprouts.
4. Heat oil in a wok and lightly stir-fry seafood for about two minutes. Remove from wok and keep warm.
5. Place stock and reserved juices in wok, add vegetables, toss, cover, and simmer for about two minutes or until vegetables are just tender and bright in colour.
6. Combine cornflour and water and mix to form a thin paste, add to vegetables and stir until sauce cooks and thickens.
7. Add drained spaghetti or noodles and seafood to vegetables, stir-fry until warmed through and serve.

NUTRITION DATA PER SERVING:
588 kcal (2465 kJ), CHO 75g, protein 48g, fat 7g.

CURRIED TUNA AND RICE CASSEROLE

SERVES FOUR

- 425g can tuna in brine
- juice of 1 lemon
- 120g basmati rice
- 2 small onions, diced
- 3 teaspoons curry powder
- 2 tablespoons flour
- 3 cups (750ml) skimmed milk
- 2 slices wholegrain bread, crumbed

⏱ 1 hour 40 minutes

VARIATION: Replace the tuna with red or pink salmon.

METHOD

1. Mix tuna and lemon juice in a bowl.
2. Cook rice in boiling water, or microwave.
3. Drain rice and combine with the tuna mixture.
4. Dry fry onion and curry powder in a saucepan.
5. Combine flour with a little of the milk to make a smooth paste.
6. Add remaining milk to onions and curry powder and bring to the boil. Remove from heat and add the flour paste.
7. Return to heat and stir continually until mixture thickens.
8. Pour two-thirds of the curry sauce over tuna and rice. Mix.
9. Spoon into a casserole and pour the remaining sauce over the top.
10. Cover with breadcrumbs, and bake in a preheated 160°C (325°F) oven until golden and the casserole is heated through (approximately 30 minutes).

NUTRITION DATA PER SERVING:
365 kcal (1527 kJ), CHO 45g, protein 36g, fat 4g.

MEATS AND POULTRY

Meats provide many essential nutrients, especially protein, Vitamin B, iron and zinc, but they can also be high in fats which is one of the reasons many people now tend to eat less meat than in the past. However, meat has been bred to be leaner over recent years. With wise shopping and low-fat cooking methods, meat can now add flavour and interest as well as valuable nutrients to meals without the disadvantages of saturated fats, which are linked to a higher risk to heart health.

Consider the cut of meat most suited to the dish you are preparing, and to the length of cooking required. The most tender cuts come from the part of the animal that has had the least exercise (near the backbone, such as fillets of beef, pork and lamb; and loin and rump cuts). These are more expensive but cook quickly and are ideal for dishes such as stir-fries. Other cuts may be tougher and need longer, moist cooking. Dishes such as curries and casseroles, which depend on long, slow cooking to develop flavour, are ideal for these cuts.

Poultry is also an excellent source of protein and other nutrients, although it is not as good a source of iron or zinc as red meat. In general the whiter cuts of poultry, such as the breast, are lower in fat than the darker meat found in the legs and wings. Under the skin is a layer of fat which can be removed with the skin. Once this is removed, poultry (apart from duck and goose) is generally a fairly low-fat meat which is versatile, absorbs flavours easily and makes an ideal basis for many dishes from different cultures.

Increasingly, many of our cooking methods and food choices are influenced by three factors. One is lack of time for food preparation, another is the influence of other cultures and cuisines, and thirdly there is a rapidly-increasing availability of prepared and semi-prepared foods in the supermarket. In addition to these changes, more and more often meat is being used as part of a dish rather than being the main component of a meal. These changes are reflected in the popularity of the stir-fry as a family meal choice, one of the easiest ways to prepare a quick, colourful and interesting meal. It can be varied to suit individual tastes and can form the basis of a vegetarian, seafood or meat meal. Just about any vegetable can be tossed in a pan or wok with a touch of oil, water or stock, garlic, herbs and spices and served with noodles or rice.

An under-used but quick and delicious meal is pancakes. On page 134 we show you how to make these and suggest some creative fillings using meat, fish or vegetables. These delectable packages can be eaten fresh or frozen and reheated at a moment's notice, adding these or many other quick and easy fillings.

STIR-FRY PORK

SERVES FOUR TO FIVE

- ◆ 500g pork fillet
- ◆ 1 tablespoon polyunsaturated oil
- ◆ ½ teaspoon grated ginger
- ◆ 1 clove garlic, crushed
- ◆ pinch Chinese five spice powder
- ◆ 1 cup (75g) small broccoli florets
- ◆ 1 cup (100g) small cauliflower florets
- ◆ ½ green capsicum (bell pepper), diced
- ◆ 2 medium carrots, cut into julienne (matchsticks)
- ◆ 3 spring onions, sliced
- ◆ 16–20 snow peas
- ◆ 10–12 button mushrooms, sliced
- ◆ 2 stalks celery, sliced diagonally
- ◆ 1 apple, cut into slices
- ◆ ¼ cucumber, cut into slices
- ◆ 1 tablespoon soy sauce
- ◆ 1 tablespoon honey
- ◆ 1 tablespoon tomato sauce
- ◆ 1½ tablespoons cornflour (cornstarch)
- ◆ 1 cup (250ml) chicken stock (see recipe, page 68)

⏱ 45 minutes

The secret of a successful stir-fry is to have all the ingredients prepared before you begin cooking, and then to cook them swiftly so that they reach the table still crisp and alive with colour.

METHOD

1. Prepare pork fillet by slicing thinly at an angle.
2. Heat oil in pan until very hot. Add pork, ginger, garlic and five spice. Stir-fry for three to five minutes.
3. Add broccoli, cauliflower, capsicum and carrots. Stir-fry for one to two minutes, making sure that nothing is allowed to over-cook and become limp.
4. Now add the rest of the vegetables and continue stir-frying over high heat for another one to two minutes.
5. In a bowl, combine soy sauce, honey, tomato sauce, cornflour and chicken stock. Add mixture to the pork and vegetables, bring to the boil, cover, turn down the heat and simmer for two to three minutes only.
6. Serve on a bed of basmati rice.

VARIATION: Replace the pork with chicken or veal.

NUTRITION DATA PER SERVING:
318 kcal (1329 kJ), CHO 25g, protein 31g, fat 11g.

PORK TANGO

SERVES FOUR

- 1 cup (250ml) boiling water
- ½ cup (85g) dried apricots
- 1 tablespoon dried currants
- 500g pork scotch fillet, trimmed of fat
- 1 beaten egg
- 2 teaspoons sesame seeds
- 2 tablespoons fresh breadcrumbs
- 1 clove garlic, finely chopped or minced (optional)
- 2 tablespoons mango chutney or fresh mango pickle (see recipe, page 172)
- 1 tablespoon brandy
- ¼ cup (60ml) canned evaporated skimmed milk

⏱ 1 hour

VARIATION: Substitute ½ cup of crushed pineapple for the apricots, but remember to reduce the water to ½ cup (125ml).

This is a favourite recipe. The brandy loses its alcohol during heating, but rounds out the lovely fruity sauce. Leave it out if you prefer.

METHOD

1. Pour boiling water over apricots and currants in a bowl, and stand for half an hour.
2. Roll pork first in egg and then in a mixture of sesame seeds, breadcrumbs and garlic until well coated.
3. Place in roasting pan and bake, uncovered, in a preheated 200°C (400°F) oven for 45 minutes.
4. While meat is cooking, heat apricots in a saucepan with the currants and the water in which they were soaked.
5. Simmer gently until water is almost absorbed.
6. Add chutney and brandy and stir until the sauce returns to the simmer.
7. Pour evaporated skimmed milk in a heat-resistant bowl and gradually stir in the hot apricot mixture (this method will prevent the milk curdling).
8. Return to saucepan and reheat without boiling.
9. To test if meat is cooked, pierce with a skewer. The juice should be clear.
10. Cut meat into eight slices, arrange two slices on each serving plate and spoon sauce over, distributing apricot halves evenly.

NUTRITION DATA PER SERVING:
252 kcal (1057 kJ), CHO 22 g, protein 34g, fat 4g.

GREEN PORK CURRY

SERVES FOUR

- 1 Spanish (red) onion, peeled and chopped
- 2 teaspoons fresh chopped ginger, or ginger paste
- 2 hot green chillies, de-seeded and chopped
- 3 tablespoons chopped fresh coriander
- grated rind and juice of 1 lime
- 1 stem fresh lemon grass, chopped, or rind of 1 lemon
- ½ teaspoon salt
- 1½ tablespoons cornflour (cornstarch)
- 1 cup (250ml) light evaporated skimmed milk
- ¾ teaspoon coconut essence
- 500g lean pork fillet, cut into bite-sized pieces
- 200g French beans, topped, tailed and halved
- ½ red capsicum (bell pepper), de-seeded and diced
- 250g bean sprouts
- sprigs of fresh basil

⏱ 35 minutes

This recipe uses evaporated skimmed milk and coconut essence instead of coconut milk—a great way to reduce the fat content! Use commercial green curry paste to make a quick but tasty meal.

METHOD

1. Blend onion, ginger, chillies, coriander, lime rind and juice, lemon grass and salt together until almost smooth. Alternatively, use 2 tablespoons of a low-fat commercial green curry paste.
2. Mix cornflour with a little evaporated milk to form a smooth paste, add remaining milk and coconut essence and set aside.
3. Spray wok with cooking oil and sauté pork until tender and just beginning to brown; set aside.
4. Add curry paste, beans and capsicum (bell pepper) to wok and toss for about two minutes.
5. Add cornflour and milk mixture and stir until sauce thickens and cooks.
6. Add bean sprouts and pork and stir until heated through.
7. Serve on bed of rice or noodles, garnished with the basil leaves.

NUTRITION DATA PER SERVING:
233 kcal (974 kJ), CHO 15g, protein 37g, fat 2g.

PORK RATATOUILLE WITH COUSCOUS

SERVES FOUR

- 2 teaspoons curry powder
- 2 tablespoons water
- 1 clove garlic, crushed
- 1 large onion, chopped
- 1 medium aubergine, chopped
- ½ medium green capsicum (bell pepper), de-seeded, chopped
- ½ medium red capsicum (bell pepper), de-seeded, chopped
- 12 small button mushrooms, washed
- 2 medium courgettes, chopped
- 800g can chopped tomatoes
- ½ cup (125ml) dry white wine (optional)
- 120g pitted black olives
- salt to taste
- 500g boneless lean pork, diced and cooked
- 2 tablespoons chopped fresh parsley
- ¾ cup (190ml) low-fat yoghurt
- 1 tablespoon cornflour (cornstarch)
- 2 cups (380g) couscous, rehydrated, to serve (see recipe, page 139)

⏲ 25 minutes

VARIATION: Replace pork with equal quantities of veal fillets.

METHOD:

1. Heat curry powder in a non-stick frying pan and add water, garlic and onion. Cook for two minutes.
2. Add the aubergine, capsicum, mushrooms and courgettes and sauté for two minutes or until softened.
3. Add the tomatoes, wine, olives and salt and bring to the boil, uncovered.
4. Reduce heat and simmer for 10 minutes or until thickened.
5. Add the pork and parsley.
6. Combine the yoghurt and cornflour, add and stir until heated through.
7. Serve over couscous.

NUTRITION DATA PER SERVING:
592 kcal (2479 kJ), CHO 65g, protein 55g, fat 10g.

MALAYSIAN FRIED RICE NOODLES (CHAR KWAY TEOW)

SERVES FOUR

- 1 tablespoon oil
- 1 clove garlic, finely chopped
- 2 small onions, cut into wedges
- 1–2 fresh chillies, deseeded and chopped
- 100g lean barbecue pork, cut into strips
- 150g green prawns, shelled and de-veined
- 150g calamari (squid) rings
- 1 cup (60g) bean sprouts
- 300g fresh rice noodles (char kway teow)
- 2 tablespoons soy sauce
- 2 teaspoons oyster sauce
- pepper to taste
- 2 eggs, beaten
- 3 spring onions, chopped, for garnish

⏱ 20 minutes

METHOD

1. Heat half the oil in a wok and fry garlic, onion and chilli until soft.
2. Add pork, prawns and calamari and continue cooking for two to three minutes or until seafood is cooked.
3. Add bean sprouts and toss.
4. Remove mixture from wok.
5. Add remaining oil to wok, heat and then add noodles. Toss gently until heated.
6. Add soy and oyster sauces and pepper and toss to mix.
7. Add eggs and stir until set.
8. Return pork and seafood mixture to wok, mix in well.
9. Serve hot garnished with chopped spring onions.

NOTE: Chinese grocery stores sell fresh rice noodles as 'sa hor fun'.

NUTRITION DATA PER SERVING:
453 kcal (1894 kJ), CHO 48g, protein 34g, fat 14g.

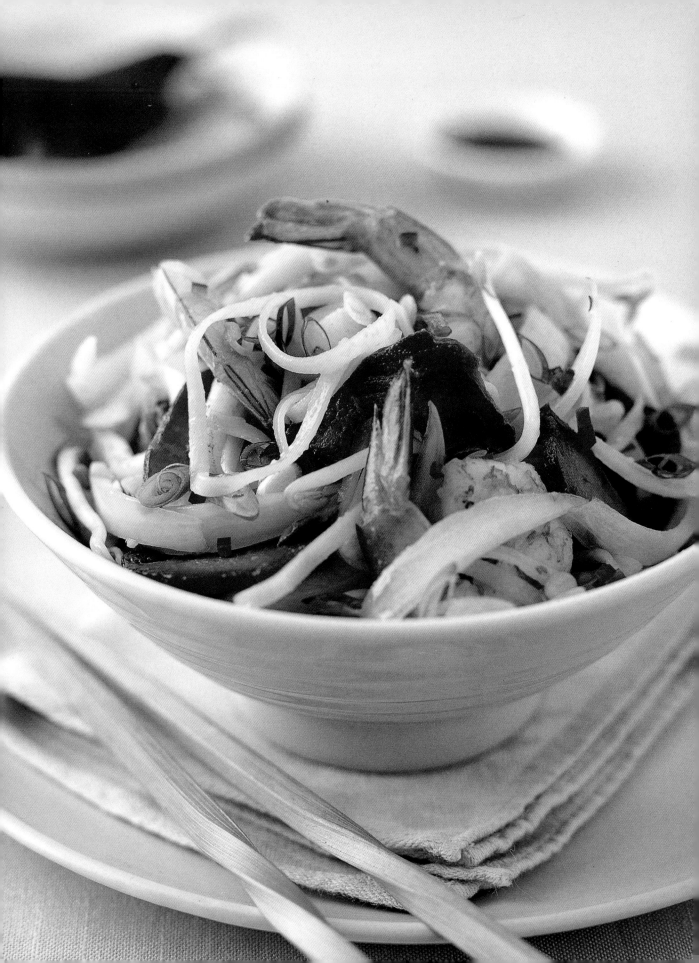

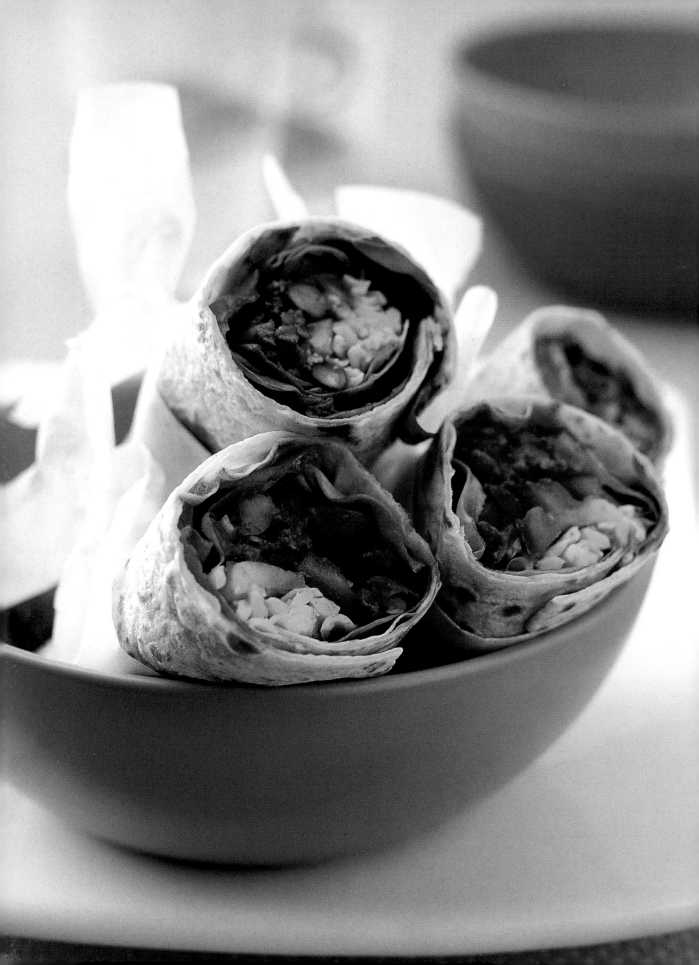

BEEF AND BEAN BURRITOS

SERVES FOUR

- ◆ 1 packet soft flour tortillas
- ◆ 500g lean minced steak
- ◆ 1 medium onion, chopped
- ◆ 1 beef stock cube or ½ teaspoon salt
- ◆ ½ teaspoon pepper
- ◆ 150g tomato purée
- ◆ 100ml water
- ◆ Tabasco sauce to taste
- ◆ juice of ½ lemon
- ◆ 410g can red kidney beans, rinsed and drained
- ◆ shredded lettuce, finely chopped onion and tomato, slices of avocado and grated low-fat cheese, to serve

⏱ 2 hours

METHOD

1. Dry fry meat until lightly browned. Add onion and continue to sauté until browned.
2. Add crumbled stock cube, pepper, tomato purée, water, sauce and lemon juice. Stir until well combined. Add kidney beans and mix in well. Bring to the boil, turn down the heat and simmer for 10–15 minutes until the meat is cooked.
3. Add extra water if necessary to make a thick sauce.
4. Keep meat and bean mixture warm until tortillas are ready or allow to cool, refrigerate and reheat when needed.
5. Heat frying pan. Place each tortilla on dry surface of frying pan. As blisters appear, press gently with egg slice or spatula. When underside is brown, turn over and cook until blisters have formed on other side and tortilla is lightly browned.
6. Lift onto tray covered with a damp tea towel. Fold tea towel to cover tortilla.
7. Repeat until all tortillas are heated through.
8. Place some hot filling onto each tortilla, together with any combination of lettuce, onion, tomato, avocado and grated cheese, and roll up. Serve immediately. Tortillas should be eaten with the fingers.

NUTRITION DATA PER SERVING (excluding raw fillings):
557 kcal (2330 kJ), CHO 75g, protein 45g, fat 8g.

MEATBALLS IN TOMATO SAUCE

SERVES FOUR

- ◆ 500g lean minced beef
- ◆ 1 tablespoon chopped parsley
- ◆ 1 teaspoon curry powder
- ◆ 3 slices wholegrain bread, crumbed
- ◆ 1 egg, beaten
- ◆ 2½ teaspoons water
- ◆ 2 medium onions, finely chopped
- ◆ 425g can tomatoes
- ◆ 1 tablespoon tomato purée
- ◆ ½ teaspoon dried oregano
- ◆ ground black pepper to taste
- ◆ chopped parsley, for garnish

🕐 1 hour 30 minutes

All you need to do is make the meatballs, prepare potatoes, brown rice, crushed wheat or noodles, make a mixed salad, and you have a perfect meal.

METHOD

1. Combine beef, parsley, curry powder and breadcrumbs in a bowl.
2. Add the egg and water to bind the mixture.
3. Roll into 16 equal balls.
4. Place in a baking dish and cook in a preheated 180°C (350°F) oven for 30 minutes. If you prefer to use the microwave, preheat a browning dish on high for six to seven minutes. Place the meatballs in the browning dish and cook on high for four to six minutes, turning the meatballs three times during the cooking process. Remove the meatballs to a shallow dish and set aside.
5. Heat saucepan with water and lightly cook the onion until translucent, stirring frequently. Alternatively, place the onions in a microwave-proof bowl and cook on high until translucent.
6. Add tomatoes, tomato purée and oregano.
7. Reduce heat and simmer for 10 minutes, or microwave on high for five minutes.
8. Add pepper to taste.
9. Pour sauce over meatballs, return to oven and reduce heat to 160°C (325°F). Bake for an additional 30 minutes. If using the microwave, cook on medium for a further 15 minutes.
10. Serve, garnished with parsley.

NUTRITION DATA PER SERVING:
243 kcal (1016 kJ), CHO 13g, protein 33g, fat 7g.

BEEF CURRY

- 500g lean beef (e.g. topside, round)
- ground black pepper
- 2 teaspoons oil (optional)
- 1 large onion, peeled and chopped
- 2 potatoes, scrubbed and chopped
- ½ cup (60g) skinned and chopped pumpkin
- ½ cup (70g) peeled and chopped sweet potato
- 2 courgettes, cut into chunks
- 1 teaspoon dried coriander
- 1 teaspoon dried cumin
- ½ teaspoon dried cardamom
- 2 teaspoons mustard seeds
- ½–1 teaspoon dried chillies
- 2 teaspoons finely chopped or minced fresh ginger
- 1 clove garlic, crushed
- 1 cup (250ml) water
- pinch of salt to taste (optional)

⏱ 2 hours 30 minutes

This dish is best when prepared the day before eating, to allow the flavour to develop. A pinch of salt helps bring out the taste of the spices, but use sparingly.

METHOD

1. Trim any fat from meat. Cut into 2–3cm (1in) cubes and sprinkle with pepper.
2. In a frying pan, dry fry meat (or sauté in 2 teaspoons of hot oil) until browned on all sides. Set aside in a bowl.
3. In the same frying pan, sauté the vegetables and set aside with the meat.
4. Add the dry spices to the frying pan and cook for three to four minutes over medium heat to release the fragrance, then add the ginger and garlic.
5. Add water and stir the pan juices well.
6. Return meat and vegetables to pan, add salt if desired, and stir to combine the flavours.
7. Spoon into a casserole, cover and cook in a preheated 200°C (400°F) oven for approximately one-and-a-half to two hours until meat is tender.
8. Serve with brown rice and an accompaniment such as fresh mango pickle (see recipe page 172), tomato mint salad (see recipe page 153), banana-yoghurt relish (see recipe page 161) or cucumber and yoghurt relish (see recipe page 161). Pineapple with paw paw, sultanas with coconut and diced apple are also excellent with curry.

NUTRITION DATA PER SERVING:
279 kcal (1169 kJ), CHO 18g, protein 31g, fat 9g.

BEEF À LA PIZZAIOLA

SERVES FOUR

- 500g lean beef fillet or rump
- 1 teaspoon oil
- 1 clove garlic, crushed
- ½ cup (35g) sliced mushrooms
- 2 large tomatoes, peeled and chopped
- 2 spring onions, chopped
- 4 leaves fresh basil, roughly chopped, or ¼ teaspoon dried basil
- freshly ground black pepper
- salt to taste (optional)
- spring onion, for garnish

⏱ 15 minutes

VARIATION: The recipe will work just as successfully if you use veal, pork or chicken. Add a few drops of Tabasco sauce if you want to make the sauce more piquant.

Although beef fillets and rumps are relatively expensive cuts of meat, in this recipe you use only 500g to feed four people. The meat cooks quickly, so there is little shrinkage and as fillet is lean, there is no waste.

METHOD

1. Cut the meat into thin strips, about 1cm x 5cm.
2. Brush oil over the base of a heavy frying pan and heat the pan over medium-high heat.
3. When hot, toss in the meat and stir-fry until well sealed and browned (approximately two to three minutes).
4. Set the meat aside on a warm plate and continue as follows. To the hot frying pan add the garlic and the mushrooms and stir-fry for a further few seconds until the mushrooms are lightly cooked.
5. Add the chopped tomatoes, spring onions, basil, pepper and salt, and bring to a simmer. Now return the meat to the sauce and simmer for about five minutes, or until the meat is cooked and the dish is hot.
6. Finally, spoon the meat and sauce onto a bed of rice or pasta, garnish with spring onion and serve.

NUTRITION DATA PER SERVING:
170 kcal (713 kJ), CHO 3g, protein 28g, fat 5g.

CORNED BEEF

- 1kg piece of beef topside
- 12 whole cloves
- 1 cup (250ml) wine vinegar (red or white)
- 1 cup (250ml) red wine
- 2 teaspoons brown sugar
- ½ teaspoon prepared mustard
- ½ teaspoon mustard seeds
- ½ teaspoon finely chopped garlic
- ½ teaspoon peppercorns
- 1 medium onion, chopped

⏱ 1 hour 30 minutes, plus 3 days marinating time

You may never have considered making your own corned beef, so this delicious recipe may be an eye-opener.

METHOD

1. Trim any fat from meat.
2. Stick cloves into meat, evenly distributed.
3. Place meat in a bowl large enough to hold it snugly.
4. Combine vinegar, wine, sugar, mustard, mustard seeds, garlic, peppercorns and onions and pour over meat.
5. Cover tightly and refrigerate for three days, turning once or twice each day.
6. Remove meat from bowl and place in large saucepan.
7. Strain marinating liquid through a sieve into smaller saucepan. Bring to boil and strain over meat.
8. Cover, bring to boil, immediately lower the heat and simmer gently until meat is cooked through (about 1 hour).
9. Serve hot with boiled or mashed potatoes and cooked red cabbage, or cold with bread or a salad.

NUTRITION DATA PER SERVING:
157 kcal (658 kJ), CHO 2g, protein 27g, fat 5g.

CHILLI CON CARNE

SERVES FOUR

- 500g beef topside
- 2 teaspoons oil (optional)
- 1 large onion, chopped
- 4 large tomatoes, chopped
- 150g can tomato purée
- 1¼ cups (300ml) water
- 425g can red kidney beans
- 1–2 teaspoons Tabasco sauce
- ¼ teaspoon ground black pepper
- 1 tablespoon cornflour (cornstarch)

⏱ 2 hours

VARIATION: This dish is equally successful if you use lean minced beef instead of topside.

METHOD

1. Trim off all fat from meat and cut into 2–3cm cubes.
2. Brush frying pan with oil and brown meat, or dry fry meat until well browned.
3. Spoon into casserole.
4. Add onion to frying pan and sauté until lightly browned.
5. Add tomatoes and cook over medium heat until soft. Stir occasionally.
6. Stir in tomato purée and 1 cup (250ml) water. Mix well.
7. Rinse kidney beans, drain well, and add to the mixture.
8. Add Tabasco sauce and pepper, pour over meat and combine.
9. Mix cornflour with remaining water. When smooth stir into mixture.
10. Cover casserole and cook in a preheated 180°C (350°F) oven until meat is tender (approximately 1½ hours).

NUTRITION DATA PER SERVING:
355 kcal (1485 kJ), CHO 34g, protein 39g, fat 7g.

STEAK WITH BLACK BEAN SAUCE

SERVES FOUR

- 2 teaspoons oil
- 500g beef fillet or lean rump steak, trimmed of fat
- 1 medium onion, peeled and quartered
- ¼ cup (30g) coarsely chopped green capsicum (bell pepper)
- ¼ cup (30g) coarsely chopped red capsicum (bell pepper)
- 1 medium carrot, sliced
- 1 quantity homemade black bean sauce (see recipe, page 165) or ½ cup (125ml) commercial sauce

🕐 30 minutes

None of the ingredients in this recipe should be cooked for more than a few minutes. At the table, the vegetables should still be crisp and retain their true vibrant colour.

METHOD

1. Brush oil over the base of a frying pan or wok and heat over high heat.
2. Slice steak into very thin strips, about 3–4cm long and 0.5cm wide. Sauté quickly for about three minutes.
3. Add vegetables and stir-fry for a further two minutes.
4. Add black bean sauce, cover and simmer gently for five minutes.
5. Serve with boiled brown rice.

NUTRITION DATA PER SERVING:
246 kcal (1031 kJ), CHO 6g, protein 32g, fat 11g.

BAKED BEEF FILLET WITH CHERRY SAUCE

SERVES EIGHT

- 1kg eye fillet of beef, trimmed of visible fat
- 2 teaspoons chopped fresh oregano or 1 teaspoon dried oregano
- 3 small sprigs fresh rosemary, or 1 teaspoon dried rosemary
- 1 quantity cherry sauce (see recipe, page 162)
- 4 sprigs oregano or rosemary, for garnish

🕐 1 hour

Eye fillet is an expensive cut, but for a special occasion it is worth it. Remember, too, that there is no waste and, in this recipe, you can serve eight with only 1kg of fillet.

METHOD

1. Place the beef on a large piece of aluminium foil.
2. Sprinkle with oregano and rosemary and wrap beef.
3. Place in a baking dish and bake for 30 minutes in a preheated 210°C (425°F) oven.
4. Uncover and bake for a further 15 minutes.
5. Remove from oven, pour juices into cherry sauce. Loosely cover meat with foil and let stand in a warm place.
6. Heat sauce.
7. Cut beef into thick slices and serve topped with cherry sauce and garnished with a sprig of oregano or rosemary.

NUTRITION DATA PER SERVING:
174 kcal (728 kJ), CHO 6g, protein 27g, fat 5g.

PASTIES

SERVES FOUR

- 200g lean minced beef
- 1 potato, finely diced
- 1 medium carrot, finely diced
- 1 small turnip, finely diced
- 1 small onion, finely diced
- ¼ teaspoon white pepper
- ¼ teaspoon dried mixed herbs
- 2 tablespoons finely chopped parsley
- 1 quantity wholemeal pastry (see recipe, page 200)
- 1 tablespoon water
- 2 tablespoons skimmed milk, for glazing

⏱ 1 hour 30 minutes

As a main course, serve pasties with vegetables and tomato and basil sauce (see recipe, page 164). They also make a wonderful light lunch meal, served with salad.

METHOD

1. In a bowl, combine meat, diced vegetables, pepper and herbs.
2. Divide pastry into four portions. Roll out each portion to about the size of a saucer.
3. Divide the meat mixture between the rounds, placing meat slightly off the centre of each round.
4. Brush the edges of the pastry with a little water. Fold pastry over in half, to make a pasty shape.
5. Use the back of a fork to crimp the edges of the pasties firmly.
6. Place the finished pasties on a lightly greased baking tray. Prick the top of each pasty three times with a fork. Brush the surface of each pasty with a little skimmed milk.
7. Bake in a preheated 200°C (400°F) oven for 35 minutes or until browned.

NUTRITION DATA PER SERVING:
567 kcal (2374 kJ), CHO 56g, protein 22g, fat 28g.

FILO ROLLS

- ◆ 200g lean minced beef
- ◆ 1 potato, finely diced
- ◆ 1 medium carrot, finely diced
- ◆ 1 small turnip, finely diced
- ◆ 1 small onion, finely diced
- ◆ ½ cup (125ml) water
- ◆ ¼ teaspoon white pepper
- ◆ ¼ teaspoon dried mixed herbs
- ◆ 2 tablespoons finely chopped parsley
- ◆ 12 sheets filo pastry
- ◆ 2 tablespoons skimmed milk, for glazing

⏱ 1 hour 20 minutes

This variation of pasties keeps the fat content down.

METHOD

1. Combine meat and vegetables in a saucepan with the water and simmer for 10 minutes. Drain.
2. Add pepper and herbs.
3. Take a sheet of filo pastry and spray with a little oil. Place another sheet on top, spray again with oil and layer one more sheet on top. Fold in half. Repeat with the remaining nine sheets of filo, so that you have four pastry rectangles.
4. Divide the meat mixture into four, place a portion on each rectangle of filo and roll into parcels. Brush the inner edges of the filo with a little semi-skimmed or skimmed milk and press down gently to seal.
5. Glaze the tops of the rolls lightly with skimmed milk. Bake in a preheated 200°C (400°F) oven for 15–20 minutes, or until crisp and lightly brown.

NUTRITION DATA PER SERVING:
205 kcal (860 kJ), CHO 28g, protein 16g, fat 3g.

MEATLOAF WITH SPICY BARBECUE SAUCE

SERVES FOUR

This meatloaf cooks in its own luscious, dark, piquant sauce.

- 500g lean minced beef
- 3 slices of wholegrain bread, crumbed
- 1 onion, finely chopped
- 2 teaspoons curry powder
- 1 tablespoon chopped parsley
- 1 egg
- ½ cup (125ml) skimmed or semi-skimmed milk
- ½ cup (125ml) water
- ½ cup (125ml) tomato sauce
- ¼ cup (60ml) Worcestershire sauce
- 2 tablespoons vinegar
- 1 teaspoon instant coffee
- juice of 1 lemon
- 1 tablespoon cornflour (cornstarch)

🕐 1 hour

METHOD

1. Combine minced beef, breadcrumbs, onion, curry powder, parsley and egg. Stir until mixture is well combined.
2. Add milk and continue stirring until mixture is smooth.
3. Shape meat mixture into a loaf and place in baking dish.
4. Bake in preheated 180°C (350°F) oven for 30 minutes, or microwave, covered, on medium for 20 minutes.
5. Remove from oven or microwave and drain off any fat.
6. In a saucepan, combine water, tomato sauce, Worcestershire sauce, vinegar, coffee and lemon juice. Bring slowly to boil, reduce heat and simmer for five minutes.
7. Pour sauce over meat and return to oven or microwave.
8. Bake for a further 20–30 minutes, basting frequently with sauce, or microwave on medium for a further 20 minutes.
9. Mix cornflour with 1 tablespoon of water to a smooth paste. Remove meatloaf to a serving plate and slice.
10. Add cornflour mixture to the sauce in the baking dish and bring back to the boil, stirring constantly until thickened.
11. Pour thickened sauce over the meatloaf. Serve hot with vegetables or cold with salad.

NUTRITION DATA PER SERVING:
289 kcal (1210 kJ), CHO 24g, protein 34g, fat 7g.

LEG OF LAMB WITH GARLIC AND MUSTARD

SERVES EIGHT

- ◆ 1.5kg leg of lamb
- ◆ 2 cloves garlic, crushed
- ◆ 1 teaspoon dried rosemary
- ◆ 2 tablespoons soy sauce
- ◆ 3 tablespoons prepared French mustard
- ◆ 2 tablespoons cornflour (cornstarch)
- ◆ 1 cup (250ml) water
- ◆ sprig of rosemary or mint, for garnish

⏱ 1–2 hours

METHOD

1. Trim all fat from the lamb and place in a baking dish.
2. Combine garlic, rosemary, soy sauce and mustard and spread over the leg of lamb.
3. Bake, covered, in a preheated 180°C (350°F) oven until cooked to your taste.
4. Remove leg of lamb from dish and carve.
5. Pour or skim the fat from meat juices.
6. Blend cornflour with a little water to form a smooth paste, and add to the meat juices.
7. Heat until thickened, stirring constantly to keep the gravy smooth, and pour over slices of lamb.

NUTRITION DATA PER SERVING:
160 kcal (671 kJ), CHO 2g, protein 27g, fat 5g.

INDIAN LAMB IN SPINACH SAUCE

SERVES FOUR

- ◆ 6 ripe tomatoes or 440g can tomatoes
- ◆ 1 tablespoon polyunsaturated vegetable oil
- ◆ 2 cloves garlic, finely chopped
- ◆ 2 teaspoons finely chopped fresh ginger
- ◆ 2 fresh green or red chillies, finely chopped, or 1 teaspoon minced chilli paste
- ◆ salt to taste
- ◆ 500g lean lamb, diced
- ◆ ¼ teaspoon each of ground cumin, coriander, cinnamon, cloves and turmeric
- ◆ 3 bunches fresh spinach, finely chopped, or 750g frozen spinach, thawed

🕐 1 hour 30 minutes

This recipe is ideal served with dry curry of potato, aubergine and pea (see recipe, page 142) and basmati rice.

METHOD

1. Blend tomatoes in a food processor.
2. Heat oil in saucepan, add garlic, ginger, chillies and salt. Cook, stirring, for two minutes.
3. Add lamb, mix well, cover and cook over low heat for 30–40 minutes or until lamb is tender.
4. Add tomatoes and cook for a further 10 minutes.
5. Add spices and simmer gently for 10 minutes.
6. Add spinach and simmer for a further four minutes.

NUTRITION DATA PER SERVING:
212 kcal (889 kJ), CHO 3g, protein 29g, fat 9g.

MOGUL LAMB

SERVES SIX

- 6 large ripe tomatoes or 440g can tomatoes, chopped
- ½ cup (125ml) water
- 4 cloves garlic, finely chopped
- 2 teaspoons finely chopped fresh ginger
- 3 fresh chillies, finely chopped
- 1 teaspoon ground black pepper
- ½ teaspoon each of ground cardamom, cloves, fennel, cinnamon and fenugreek
- 4 tablespoons chopped fresh coriander leaves
- 1 tablespoon each of chopped fresh basil, dill and mint
- salt to taste
- 1 x 1.5kg leg of lamb, boned and trimmed of all visible fat

⏱ 1 hour 45 minutes

METHOD

1. Place tomatoes, water, garlic, ginger, chillies and pepper into a saucepan and simmer, stirring occasionally for 15 minutes.
2. Add all other ingredients but the lamb, mix well and set aside.
3. Place lamb into a casserole dish, spread well with tomato mixture, cover and stand for 20 minutes in refrigerator to marinate.
4. Place, uncovered, in a preheated 180°C (350°F) oven and bake for 1 hour 15 minutes or until cooked.
5. Serve accompanied with spiced rice with peas (see recipe, page 146).

VARIATION: Use 1kg lean diced lamb or fillets and reduce cooking time accordingly.

NUTRITION DATA PER SERVING:
213 kcal (891 kJ), CHO 2g, protein 37g, fat 6g.

VEAL MANGO

SERVES FOUR

- ◆ 2 small or 1 large mango
- ◆ 1 cup (250ml) dry white wine
- ◆ 3 tablespoons mango chutney or fresh mango pickle (see recipe, page 172)
- ◆ 4 tablespoons chopped spring onions
- ◆ 4 lean veal schnitzels
- ◆ a little plain flour
- ◆ 1 teaspoon oil
- ◆ 2 tablespoons water
- ◆ 4 spring onions, for garnish

⏱ 40 minutes

This is a wonderful recipe that is very easy to prepare and yet looks and tastes good enough for a special occasion. Simple boiled rice and a crisp green salad round out the meal. Pork schnitzel or chicken fillets make an excellent and economical substitute for the veal.

METHOD

1. Make the sauce. Peel the mangoes. Cut away and roughly slice the flesh.
2. Place the mango flesh in a saucepan. Add the white wine and pickle or chutney. Bring to the boil, reduce heat and simmer until the sauce has reduced by half, about 15 minutes.
3. If you want a smooth sauce, purée the hot fruit mixture in a food processor or blender, or force through a sieve. Return to saucepan.
4. Add the chopped spring onions. Return to the boil, reduce heat and simmer for a further two to three minutes.
5. Dust the veal schnitzels with the plain flour. While the sauce is simmering, brush or spray a large frying pan with oil and heat over medium-high heat.
6. Fry the schnitzels, turning occasionally, for approximately 10 minutes until browned on both sides.
7. Remove the cooked schnitzels from the pan. Add the 2 tablespoons of water to the pan, as well as the sauce. Heat, stirring constantly, for about three minutes.
8. Arrange the schnitzels on individual dinner plates. Spoon the sauce over the schnitzels and garnish with the whole spring onions.

NUTRITION DATA PER SERVING:
175 kcal (734 kJ), CHO 9g, protein 28g, fat 3g.

CHICKEN ENCHILADAS

SERVES FOUR

- 2 cups (280g) cooked, chopped skinless chicken breast
- 1 small onion, finely chopped
- 8–10 drops Tabasco sauce or to taste
- ¼ teaspoon salt
- ¼ teaspoon ground black pepper
- 8 soft flour tortillas, suitable for enchiladas
- 2 cups (500ml) fresh tomato purée or commercial pasta sauce
- additional Tabasco sauce to taste
- ½ cup (60g) grated reduced-fat cheddar cheese
- 1 ripe avocado
- juice ½ lemon

🕐 1 hour

Don't try storing the enchiladas, they will become soggy. You should serve them immediately they are heated through. Heat them in the oven, not in the microwave.

METHOD

1. Combine chicken and onion in a mixing bowl.
2. Add Tabasco sauce, salt and pepper, to chicken mixture. Mix well. Taste and adjust seasoning.
3. Preheat tortillas in oven or microwave to soften.
4. Wrap each tortilla around one eighth of chicken mixture. Pack into casserole or baking dish.
5. Combine tomato purée with Tabasco sauce, and pour over chicken rolls.
6. Sprinkle with cheese.
7. Bake in a preheated 200°C (400°F) oven until rolls are heated through and cheese has melted.
8. Peel avocado and remove stone. Mash flesh in a separate bowl with lemon juice.
9. Spoon a little avocado mixture over each serving.

NUTRITION DATA PER SERVING:
486 kcal (2033 kJ), CHO 26g, protein 39g, fat 25g.

CHICKEN WITH STRAWBERRY AND PEPPERCORN SAUCE

SERVES FOUR

- ◆ 2 teaspoons oil
- ◆ 4 chicken fillets
- ◆ 1 quantity strawberry and peppercorn sauce (see recipe, page 166)

⏱ 15 minutes

Some unusual combinations don't quite make the mark, but this one is delicious and worthy of a special occasion.

METHOD

1. Brush the frying pan with oil and heat over medium heat. Sauté the chicken fillets until cooked and golden brown. (You can microwave them on high for three minutes but they will not brown.)
2. Prepare sauce as described on page 166.
3. Arrange fillets on serving plates, spoon over the sauce and serve accompanied by blanched green beans.

VARIATION: Sliced turkey breast with strawberry and peppercorn sauce makes a wonderful Christmas dinner.

NUTRITION DATA PER SERVING:
237 kcal (922 kJ), CHO 7g, protein 30g, fat 8g.

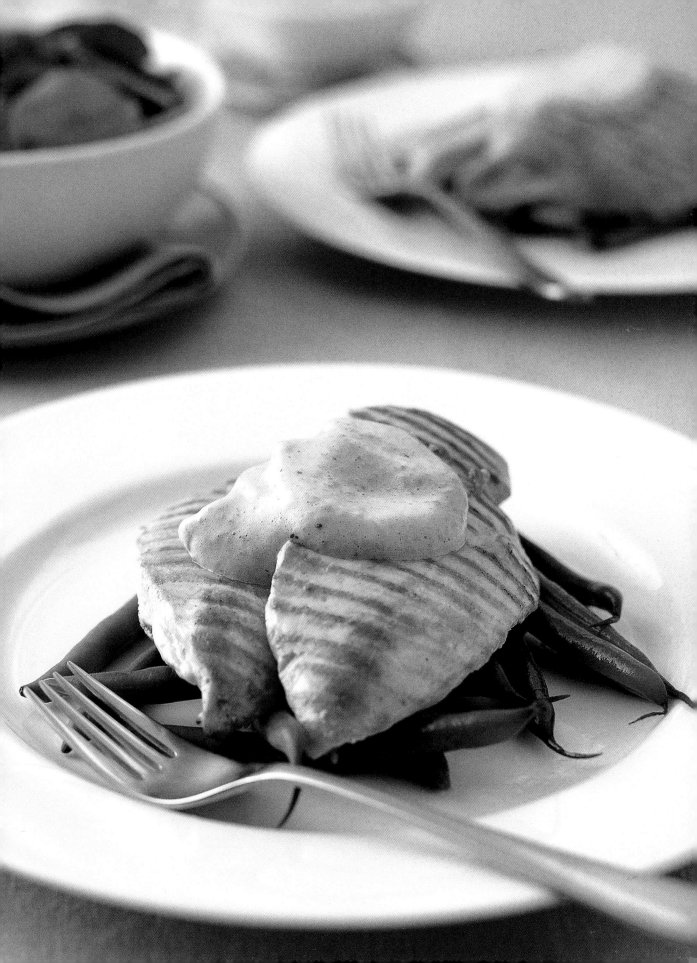

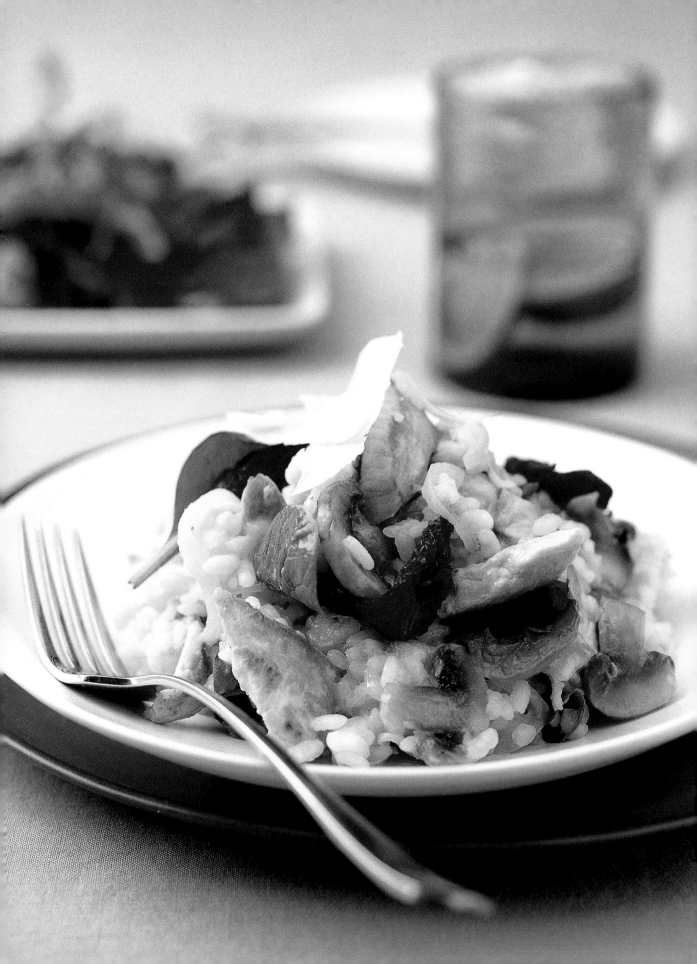

CHICKEN, SUN-DRIED TOMATO AND MUSHROOM RISOTTO

SERVES FOUR

- 2 cloves garlic, finely chopped
- 1 medium onion, peeled and sliced
- 4 cups (1 litre) chicken stock
- 2 cups (410g) arborio rice, well washed
- 2 large chicken fillets, cut into bite-size pieces
- ½ cup (40g) sun-dried tomatoes, cut in half
- 1 cup (70g) button mushrooms
- black pepper, to taste
- 1 cup (35g) baby spinach leaves
- 2 rounded tablespoons ricotta cheese
- 2 tablespoons freshly grated parmesan cheese

⏱ 20 minutes

SEAFOOD VARIATION: Replace chicken and sun-dried tomatoes with 2 cups mixed seafood (white fish, prawns, scallops, mussels, crab meat and/or oysters). Sprinkle with chopped parsley.

ITALIAN VARIATION: During cooking add 4 diced anchovy fillets, ¼ cup pitted olives and 1 tablespoon of capers. Replace spinach with ½ cup chopped peeled tomatoes.

METHOD

1. In a large saucepan, sauté garlic, onion and chicken pieces in a little stock and set aside.
2. Place remainder of stock in saucepan and bring to boil.
3. Add ½ cup rice and gently stir until stock boils again.
4. Add a further ½ cup of rice and stir till stock boils again.
5. Repeat until all the rice is added to pan.
6. Add the chicken mixture, tomatoes, mushrooms and black pepper.
7. Reduce heat and cook gently, stirring occasionally, for about 15 minutes until the rice is cooked and all the stock absorbed.
8. Add spinach and toss to allow leaves to wilt.
9. Remove risotto from heat and stir in ricotta cheese.
10. Serve on individual plates and sprinkle with parmesan cheese.

NUTRITION DATA PER SERVING:
476 kcal (1996 kJ), CHO 83g, protein 24g, fat 5g.

GOLDEN CHICKEN RISOTTO

SERVES FOUR

- 2 tablespoons water
- 1 large onion, chopped
- 1 clove garlic, crushed
- 1½ cups (300g) basmati rice
- 6 cups (1½ litres) chicken stock
  or 4 chicken stock cubes dissolved
  in 6 cups (1½ litres) water
- 4 skinless chicken breasts, finely diced
- 1 teaspoon powdered turmeric
- 20 almonds, blanched and halved
- 3 tablespoons raisins

⏱ 1 hour

There are two ways of preparing this dish—on top of the stove or in the oven. They are equally effective. Serve the risotto hot, accompanied by a green salad.

METHOD

1. If cooking the risotto in the oven, place all ingredients in a casserole. Cover and cook in a preheated 180°C (350°F) oven for one hour, or until rice has absorbed the stock and is tender.
2. For the stovetop version, boil the water in a saucepan, add the onion and cook until softened.
3. Add the garlic and cook for two minutes.
4. Add the rice and one quarter of the chicken stock. Bring to the boil. Reduce heat and simmer for 20 minutes, stirring occasionally and adding more stock, as necessary, to prevent sticking.
5. Add the diced chicken breasts, turmeric, almonds and raisins.
6. Continue simmering a further 20–25 minutes, adding remaining stock as necessary, until the rice is tender. There should be no liquid in the finished risotto.

NUTRITION DATA PER SERVING:
488 kcal (2044 kJ), CHO 65g, protein 32g, fat 11g.

CHICKEN TIKKA

SERVES FOUR

- 200g low-fat natural yoghurt
- juice 1 lemon
- 1 teaspoon finely chopped or minced ginger
- 1 teaspoon finely chopped or minced garlic
- ¼ teaspoon dried coriander
- ½ teaspoon powdered turmeric
- 2 tablespoons chopped fresh mint
- ¼ teaspoon ground black pepper
- ¼ teaspoon garam masala
- 4 skinless chicken breasts or thighs

⏱ 2 hours

This is simple to make and superbly fragrant. All you need to add is plenty of carbohydrate-rich accompaniments and steamed vegetables or a crisp salad.

METHOD
1. Combine yoghurt, lemon juice and flavourings in a bowl.
2. Add chicken and cover well with marinade. Cover and marinate for two to three hours.
3. Lift chicken from marinade. Place on baking dish. Cover with aluminium foil and bake in a preheated 200°C (400°F) oven for 30 minutes.
4. Remove foil, spoon remaining marinade over and bake until chicken is tender and lightly browned (½–1 hour).

NUTRITION DATA PER SERVING:
173 kcal (723 kJ), CHO 4g, protein 27g, fat 6g.

CHICKEN SOY

SERVES FOUR

- 4 spring onions, sliced
- 2 cloves garlic, crushed
- 2 teaspoons grated fresh ginger
- ⅓ cup (80ml) soy sauce
- 3 tablespoons dry sherry
- 4 skinless chicken breasts
- chopped parsley, chives or spring onions, for garnish

⏱ 3 hours

VARIATION: Try a garnish of three tablespoons of sesame seeds added before baking instead of the garnish suggested in the recipe.

METHOD
1. Prepare the marinade. In a bowl, combine all the ingredients, except the chicken.
2. Arrange the chicken breasts in a baking dish. Pour over the marinade. Cover with plastic film and refrigerate for two hours, turning occasionally.
3. Bake them, uncovered, in a preheated 180°C (350°F) oven for 40 minutes, basting occasionally, or cover and microwave on medium for 20–25 minutes.
4. Remove chicken from baking dish and arrange on a serving platter. Brush with pan juices. Sprinkle with chopped parsley, chives or spring onions.

NUTRITION DATA PER SERVING:
164 kcal (685 kJ), CHO 3g, protein 26g, fat 5g.

FIVE-SPICE CHICKEN

SERVES FOUR

- ¼ teaspoon Chinese five-spice powder
- ½ teaspoon chilli powder (or to taste)
- 1 teaspoon soy sauce
- 1 clove garlic, crushed
- ¾ cup (750g) low-fat natural yoghurt
- 4 skinless chicken breasts

⏱ 1 hour 15 minutes plus 4 hours marinating time

METHOD

1. Fold five-spice powder, chilli powder, soy sauce and garlic gently into yoghurt.
2. Coat chicken breasts in yoghurt mixture and allow to stand for at least four hours.
3. Place in shallow casserole, cover with lid or aluminium foil, and bake for an hour in a preheated low to moderate 150°C (300°F) oven or until tender, turning occasionally.

NUTRITION DATA PER SERVING:
176 kcal (736 kJ), CHO 4g, protein 28g, fat 6g.

APRICOT CHICKEN

SERVES FOUR

- 2 cups (460g) solid-pack canned apricots
- 4 skinless chicken breasts
- 1 large onion, chopped coarsely
- ground black pepper, to taste
- 2 sage leaves, finely chopped or ½ teaspoon dried sage
- 1 sprig thyme, chopped
- 1 tablespoon fruit chutney
- 1 tablespoon cornflour (cornstarch)
- 2 tablespoons water
- 1 tablespoon finely chopped chives or mint, for garnish

⏱ 40 minutes

METHOD

1. Reserve four apricot halves for garnish. Purée remaining apricots in a food processor or blender or press through a sieve.
2. Arrange chicken fillets in a single layer in a casserole. Sprinkle over onion, pepper and herbs.
3. Combine chutney and apricot purée and pour over the chicken. Bake in a preheated 180°C (350°F) oven for 30 minutes.
4. Mix the cornflour and water to a smooth paste.
5. Remove casserole from oven. Use a slotted spoon to lift out chicken breasts; cover and keep warm.
6. Drain the sauce from the casserole into a saucepan. Add the cornflour paste to the sauce and heat, stirring constantly, until it thickens. Cook a further two minutes.
7. Arrange a chicken breast on each plate and spoon sauce over each one. Garnish with apricot halves and chopped chives and serve.

NUTRITION DATA PER SERVING:
192 kcal (805 kJ), CHO 11g, protein 26g, fat 5g.

SATAY CHICKEN

SERVES FOUR (3 skewers each)

- ◆ 500g chicken fillets
- ◆ 1 clove garlic, crushed
- ◆ 2 tablespoons soy sauce
- ◆ 2 tablespoons lemon juice
- ◆ 1 small onion, grated
- ◆ 1 teaspoon oil

⏱ 1 hour 30 minutes

A Malaysian recipe that makes a great alternative for the barbecue. Green prawns, pork, beef or lamb fillet are all delicious cooked with this marinade.

METHOD

1. Soak 12 wooden skewers in water for at least an hour, to prevent them burning on the barbecue.
2. Cut chicken into small cubes.
3. Thread the chicken onto skewers. Arrange the skewers on a flat dish.
4. Combine remaining ingredients and brush over the chicken. Leave chicken to marinate for at least an hour, turning occasionally.
5. Grill or barbecue the satay chicken, turning frequently and basting from time to time with marinade.
6. Serve hot, accompanied by peanut sauce (see recipe, page 163), gado gado (see recipe, page 125) and brown rice.

NUTRITION DATA PER SERVING:
169 kcal (708 kJ), CHO 1g, protein 26g, fat 7g.

CHICKEN WITH MUSTARD SEED SAUCE

SERVES FOUR

- 4 chicken fillets, skinless
- ½ cup (125ml) tomato sauce
- 1 teaspoon Tabasco sauce
- 2 tablespoons seeded mustard
- 1 tablespoon Worcestershire sauce
- 1 tablespoon brown vinegar
- 1 clove garlic, crushed

⏱ 1 hour

This is so easy to make and, once it's in the oven, you don't need to think about it again until you're ready to bring it to the table.

METHOD

1. Arrange chicken in casserole.
2. Combine tomato sauce, Tabasco sauce, mustard, Worcestershire sauce, vinegar and garlic.
3. Pour over chicken.
4. Cover and bake in a preheated 180°C (350°F) oven for 45 minutes. Alternatively, cover and microwave on medium for 35 minutes.
5. Serve with cooked rice and hot vegetables or salad.

NUTRITION DATA PER SERVING:
179 kcal (749 kJ), CHO 3g, protein 26g, fat 7g.

DRUNKEN RABBIT CASSEROLE

SERVES FOUR

- 800g rabbit, jointed
- 1 teaspoon vinegar or lemon juice
- 1 medium onion, sliced
- 1 cup (250ml) water
- ½ cup (125ml) red wine
- 2 chicken stock cubes, crumbled
- 1 tablespoon tomato purée
- 2 medium tomatoes, chopped
- ½ teaspoon dried oregano
- 6 spring onions, chopped
- 16 small button mushrooms or canned champignons
- 1 tablespoon cornflour (cornstarch)
- 1 tablespoon water

⏱ 2 hours 15 minutes

VARIATION: If rabbit is unavailable, you can use lean chicken instead. You'll need about 500g of chicken breast.

METHOD

1. Soak rabbit in cold water with vinegar or lemon juice for 30 minutes. Discard water.
2. In a casserole, combine the rabbit, onion, water, wine, stock cubes, tomato purée, chopped tomatoes and oregano. Cover and bake in a preheated 180°C (350°F) oven for 1¼ hours, or microwave on medium for 30–40 minutes.
3. Remove casserole from oven. Add the spring onions and mushrooms and stir. Cover, return to oven and bake for a further 15 minutes or microwave on high for five minutes.
4. Remove casserole from oven. Using a slotted spoon, lift the rabbit and vegetables onto a serving platter, cover and keep warm.
5. Pour the juices into a saucepan.
6. In a cup, mix the cornflour and water to make a smooth paste and add to the cooking juices. Bring to the boil, stirring constantly, until thickened. Reduce heat and simmer for two minutes.
7. Pour the sauce over the rabbit and vegetables and serve at once.

NUTRITION DATA PER SERVING:
238 kcal (997 kJ), CHO 12g, protein 30g, fat 8g.

SWEET AND SOUR RABBIT WITH PRUNES

- 800g rabbit, jointed
- 1 cup (250ml) dry white wine
- 2 medium onions, sliced
- 1½ cups (375ml) chicken stock (see recipe, page 68) or 1½ cups (375ml) water and 2 chicken stock cubes
- 1 bay leaf
- 1 tablespoon redcurrant jelly
- 6–8 peppercorns, according to taste
- 8 whole prunes, stoned
- ¼ cup (40g) seedless raisins
- 2 tablespoon cornflour (cornstarch)
- 1 tablespoon vinegar
- freshly milled black pepper
- chopped parsley, for garnish

⏲ 2 hours plus overnight soaking time

Rabbit is low in fat and easy to prepare.

METHOD

1. Marinate rabbit overnight in the wine and onions.
2. Discard the onions, place the rabbit and wine marinade in a flameproof casserole, and add the chicken stock, bay leaf, redcurrant jelly and peppercorns and bring to the boil. Turn down the heat.
3. Add the prunes and raisins; submerge them in the cooking liquid, cover the casserole tightly and bake in a preheated 160°C (325°F) oven for about 1½ hours until the rabbit is tender and the prunes are plump.
4. Remove from oven, lift out the rabbit and remove the bones. Set meat aside and strain the cooking juices into a clean pan, retaining the prunes and raisins.
5. Blend cornflour with vinegar to form a smooth paste, add to juices and boil for one to two minutes, stirring all the time until the sauce thickens. Arrange the rabbit, prunes and raisins in the casserole and pour the thickened juices over. Garnish with parsley and black pepper.

NUTRITION DATA PER SERVING:
275 kcal (1152 kJ), CHO 17g, protein 32g, fat 9g.

MEATLESS DISHES

There are many people who choose a vegetarian style of eating, or who regularly enjoy meatless meals. This style of cooking fits in well with the principles of healthy eating for people with diabetes. However, if you choose a completely vegetarian way of eating, you do need to make sure you balance your meals well to ensure all your nutrient needs are met. On pages 46–47 we show you how to do this.

Many non-meat meals have the advantage of providing carbohydrate as well as protein. If prepared with the minimum of added fats and oils, they can also be low in fat, and are often cheaper than their meat-based counterparts. Do remember that the addition of cheese, creams, butter, margarine and oils adds to the total fat content, so use them sparingly, or try many of the low-fat alternatives now available. In our recipes you will find these principles are followed with delicious results. We have included a wide range of meatless dishes for you to try which contain pulses, pasta, rice, nuts and seeds, or eggs, tofu and reduced-fat cheese.

Pulses (dried beans, peas and lentils) provide an excellent source of protein, carbohydrate, iron and fibre, as well as useful amounts of calcium, potassium and B-vitamins. Their other advantage is their low glycaemic index, a plus for people with diabetes. Most pulses need soaking and long, slow cooking to make them soft and digestible which means planning ahead. They can, however, be cooked ahead of time, divided into portions and frozen, then thawed for use in quick and tasty meals. Many pulse-based dishes also freeze well, so can simply be reheated and served. To save time for the busy family cook, it is now easy to buy a wide range of canned pulses already cooked and ready to add to recipes.

Nuts and seeds are useful additions to dishes for flavour and texture as well as nutrition. They are, however, fairly high in fat, so use in moderation. Eggs, tofu and reduced-fat cheeses are excellent sources of protein and other important nutrients, but are low in carbohydrate. You will find many of our recipes show you how to combine these nutritious ingredients with the carbohydrates (including rice, pastas, pulses and couscous) needed for energy during the day.

JUMPING BEAN BAKE

SERVES FOUR

- ◆ 2 cups (380g) dried beans (any variety), or 4 cups (720g) canned and drained beans such as lima, borlotti, kidney, soy or haricot
- ◆ 1 cup (250ml) tomato purée
- ◆ ¼ teaspoon cayenne pepper
- ◆ 2 cloves garlic, crushed
- ◆ 1 teaspoon dried oregano
- ◆ 1 bay leaf
- ◆ 500g ripe tomatoes, sliced
- ◆ 2 medium onions, sliced
- ◆ ½ cup (30g) fresh wholegrain breadcrumbs
- ◆ 4 tablespoons grated, reduced-fat cheddar cheese

🕐 2 hours 15 minutes plus overnight soaking of beans

VARIATION: For a thicker version of this dish, mash half the beans and leave the rest whole at the end of step three.

METHOD

1. Place dried beans in a saucepan, cover with water and soak overnight (do not soak the beans in an aluminium saucepan).
2. Drain the beans and rinse them thoroughly in cold water.
3. Return beans to the saucepan and cover with fresh water. Bring to boil, reduce heat and simmer, loosely covered, for one hour or until tender, or microwave on high for 5 minutes, then medium–low for 30 minutes or until tender. Drain beans, discarding water.
4. If you are using canned beans, drain and rinse well.
5. In a bowl, combine the tomato purée, cayenne pepper, garlic and herbs.
6. Lightly grease the casserole, and place a layer of beans on the base, cover with a layer of tomatoes and then a layer of onions. Repeat the layers until all the ingredients are used.
7. Pour tomato mixture over, top with breadcrumbs and cheese.
8. Cover and bake in a preheated 180°C (350°F) oven for one hour, then remove cover and bake for another hour or until beans start to break apart. Alternatively, cover and microwave on medium for 45 minutes, then remove the cover and microwave for another 30 minutes or until the beans start to break apart.
9. Serve immediately.

NUTRITION DATA PER SERVING:
382 kcal (1601 kJ), CHO 55g, protein 29g, fat 4g.

VEGETABLE LOAF

SERVES SIX

- ◆ 2 tablespoons water
- ◆ 2 medium onions, chopped
- ◆ 2 sticks celery, chopped
- ◆ ½ green capsicum (bell pepper), chopped
- ◆ 2 teaspoons curry powder
- ◆ ½ cup (120g) cooked potato, mashed
- ◆ ½ cup (85g) cooked pumpkin, mashed
- ◆ 1 cup (250g) ricotta cheese
- ◆ 1 cup (140g) coarsely ground cashew nuts
- ◆ ½ cup (45g) rolled oats
- ◆ 2 tablespoons chopped parsley
- ◆ 1 teaspoon chopped fresh thyme or ½ teaspoon dried thyme
- ◆ 2 tablespoons sesame seeds
- ◆ 1 quantity cheese sauce (see recipe, page 163), or fresh vegetable sauce (see recipe, page 164)

⏱ 1 hour

This loaf is very high in fibre, and is delicious eaten hot or cold with one of the sauces we recommend.

METHOD

1. In a frying pan, or in a bowl in the microwave, heat the water and sauté onions, celery, capsicum and curry powder for three minutes.
2. In a bowl, combine the sautéed vegetables with the rest of the ingredients.
3. Line a loaf tin with foil and spray with spray oil.
4. Sprinkle sesame seeds over base of tin, and then shake tin so that seeds adhere to sides as well.
5. Spoon vegetable mixture into the tin and press down firmly and neatly.
6. Bake in a preheated 180°C (350°F) oven for 40 minutes.
7. Remove from oven and leave to stand for five minutes before turning out. Turn onto serving dish and carefully remove foil.
8. Finally, grill on high for three to five minutes or until the top is crisp and well browned.
9. To serve: cut loaf into thick slices, but do not separate them, then spoon over the hot sauce.

NUTRITION DATA PER SERVING:
425 kcal (1781 kJ), CHO 25g, protein 29g, fat 24g.

VEGETARIAN LASAGNE

SERVES FOUR TO SIX

- a little oil
- 2 medium onions, peeled and chopped
- 3 large tomatoes, chopped
- 150g tomato purée
- 2 cups (500ml) water
- 1–2 teaspoons crushed or finely chopped garlic
- 1 teaspoon dried mixed herbs
- ¼ teaspoon black pepper
- ¼ teaspoon salt
- 750g can three-bean mix or kidney beans
- 250g frozen spinach
- 9 sheets instant lasagne
- ½ cup (60g) grated reduced-fat cheddar cheese
- 2 tablespoons grated parmesan cheese
- ½ cup (100g) cottage cheese

⏱ 2 hours

This dish is even better if prepared the day before it is to be served, so that the flavour can fully develop. It freezes well, so prepare a few and store them in the freezer as a standby.

METHOD

1. Wipe or spray a frying pan with oil, heat it and sauté onions until lightly browned, stirring to prevent burning.
2. Add tomatoes and cook for about five minutes until soft.
3. Add tomato purée and water and mix thoroughly.
4. Add seasonings.
5. Rinse and drain beans and add to tomato mixture. Combine well.
6. Simmer gently, covered, until you are ready to assemble the lasagne. If sauce becomes too thick, add a little water.
7. Place spinach in saucepan. Cook very gently, uncovered, until it is fairly dry.
8. Spoon a thin layer of tomato and bean sauce over base of dish.
9. Arrange a layer of lasagne on top.
10. Spoon on more sauce, sprinkle with half the reduced-fat cheese and half the parmesan.
11. Top with another layer of lasagne and cover this with spinach, cottage cheese and the remaining parmesan.
12. Place the last layer of lasagne over this, cover with the remaining sauce and, lastly, sprinkle with the remaining grated, reduced-fat cheese.
13. Cover with foil and bake in a preheated 180°C (350°F) oven for 30 minutes. Remove the foil, and bake for a further 30 minutes or until lasagne is tender.

NUTRITION DATA PER SERVING:
327 kcal (1369 kJ), CHO 42g, protein 25g, fat 6g.

CHEESE AND SPINACH ROLLS

SERVES FOUR

- 1 bunch fresh spinach or 250g packet frozen spinach
- 2 tablespoons water
- 4 spring onions, chopped
- 1 cup (250g) ricotta cheese
- 1 cup (190g) cooked basmati rice
- 2 tablespoons lemon juice
- pinch nutmeg
- 12 sheets filo pastry
- spray oil

🕐 45 minutes

VARIATION: Try adding 2 tablespoons of pine nuts or chopped walnuts to the filling mixture.

Serve these fragrant rolls with cheese sauce (see recipe, page 163) spooned over them.

METHOD

1. Wash fresh spinach very thoroughly under cold, running water. Do not dry it. Chop roughly. Place wet, chopped spinach in a large saucepan. Cover and cook over high heat for about 10 minutes or until tender. Remove spinach from saucepan and drain well. Set aside to cool. (If you use frozen spinach, cook it uncovered in a saucepan over low heat until excess water has evaporated; set aside to cool.)
2. Bring water to the boil in a saucepan, add the spring onions and cook until softened.
3. Combine onions with spinach, cheese, rice, lemon juice and nutmeg and blend well.
4. Fold a sheet of filo pastry in half widthwise. Spray lightly with oil. Repeat with another two sheets of filo. Place them on top of the first sheet, and spray each sheet with oil. You now have six layers of pastry.
5. Place a quarter of the filling along the edge of the pastry and roll up to encase the filling. Lift and tuck in the ends of the pastry before the last roll. This makes a neat parcel.
6. Place the completed roll, seal-side down, on a lightly greased baking tray.
7. Repeat steps four to six to make four cheese and spinach rolls.
8. Spray each roll with oil. Bake in a preheated 200°C (400°F) oven for 15 minutes or until pastry is crisp and golden.

NUTRITION DATA PER SERVING:
272 kcal (1139 kJ), CHO 37g, protein 14g, fat 7g.

TIBETAN PIE

- 1 quantity wholemeal pastry (see recipe, page 200)
- 500g frozen spinach
- 6 medium potatoes, washed but not peeled and cut into large pieces
- 1 large onion, chopped
- 4 tablespoons chopped fresh mixed herbs (e.g. mint, thyme, parsley, oregano, marjoram)
- ½ teaspoon coarsely ground black pepper
- 1 teaspoon salt (optional)
- ½ teaspoon nutmeg
- 1 teaspoon curry powder
- 2 teaspoons margarine

⏱ 1 hour 30 minutes

Keep pastry cool in the refrigerator while preparing the filling; this prevents the pastry from becoming soggy when you add hot filling.

METHOD

1. Cook spinach in saucepan until excess water has evaporated. The spinach should be fairly dry.
2. Boil potatoes until tender. Drain and mash potatoes roughly so that some pieces remain.
3. Add spinach, onion, herbs, spices and margarine.
4. Cut off two-thirds of the pastry and roll out to cover the base and sides of a pie dish.
5. Spoon filling onto pastry, brush pastry edge with a little water.
6. Roll out the remaining pastry. Place on top of filling. Pierce the top of the pastry with a fork.
7. Trim the pastry to size and pinch the edges of pastry together.
8. Bake in a preheated 200°C (400°F) oven for approximately 45 minutes or until lightly browned.

NUTRITION DATA PER SERVING:
424 kcal (1776 kJ), CHO 50g, protein 12g, fat 19g.

MEXICALE PIE WITH POLENTA DUMPLINGS

SERVES FOUR

- 2 teaspoons oil
- 1 finely chopped onion
- 2 cloves garlic, crushed
- 1 green capsicum (bell pepper), diced
- 2 tablespoons tomato purée
- 440g can whole tomatoes
- 440g can corn kernels, drained
- 780g can kidney beans, drained
- ½ teaspoon allspice
- 1 teaspoon chilli powder, or to taste
- 1 bay leaf
- 2 teaspoons Worcestershire sauce
- ½ cup (125ml) water
- 1 cup (140g) wholemeal self-raising flour
- 1 cup (150g) polenta (cornmeal)
- ¾ cup (190ml) semi-skimmed milk
- 2 eggs, lightly beaten
- 1 cup (120g) grated reduced-fat cheddar cheese
- 2 tablespoons chopped chives

⏱ 1 hour 15 minutes

The dumplings give this already nutritious and flavoursome dish an extra carbohydrate punch. Experiment with the flavourings according to your taste for spicy food. We have suggested canned vegetables and beans to make the dish quick to prepare.

METHOD

1. Heat oil in the saucepan over medium heat and then sauté onion, garlic and capsicum for approximately three minutes until just tender.
2. Add tomato purée, vegetables, spices, bay leaf, Worcestershire sauce and water.
3. Boil, uncovered, for 15 minutes, then remove bay leaf.
4. Transfer bean mixture to baking dish or casserole.
5. Make the dumplings by combining the flour, cornmeal, milk, eggs, cheese and chives. Drop spoonfuls of dumpling mixture on top of the bean mixture.
6. Bake, uncovered, in a preheated 200°C (400°F) oven for 10 minutes, then reduce heat to 180°C (350°F) and bake for a further 30 minutes. Serve hot.

NUTRITION DATA PER SERVING:
755 kcal (3160 kJ), CHO 99g, protein 48g, fat 17g.

BOMBAY BURGERS WITH CUCUMBER AND YOGHURT SAUCE

SERVES FOUR

(makes eight patties)

- 1 cup (190g) dried red lentils
- 1 large potato, cut into pieces
- 1 medium onion, finely chopped
- ¼ cup (20g) shredded coconut
- 1 tablespoon sesame seeds
- 1 tablespoon plain flour
- 1 teaspoon curry powder
- 1 teaspoon finely chopped
  fresh ginger
- ½ teaspoon salt
- ¼ teaspoon pepper
- 2 teaspoons lemon juice
- ¾–1 cup (55–75g) wheatgerm or
  wholegrain breadcrumbs
- sliced onion rings, for garnish
- 1 quantity of cucumber and yoghurt
  sauce (see recipe, page 166)

🕐 1 hour

METHOD

1. Soak lentils in water for 2 hours.
2. Rinse, cover with water in a saucepan and simmer for approximately 30 minutes until tender.
3. Add potato 10 minutes into the cooking time. Alternatively, place lentils in a bowl with water and microwave on high for 20 minutes or until tender. Add potato 10 minutes into the cooking time.
4. Drain any liquid from lentils and potato, and mash thoroughly. Add onion, coconut, sesame seeds, flour, spices and lemon juice.
5. Allow to cool (preferably chill).
6. Shape into patties and coat with wheatgerm or breadcrumbs.
7. Bake on lightly oiled tray in a preheated 190°C (375°F) oven for 10–15 minutes, or cook in a frying pan lightly brushed with oil, taking care not to burn the coating.
8. Serve hot garnished with onion rings and with cucumber and yoghurt sauce.

NUTRITION DATA PER SERVING:
200 kcal (838 kJ), CHO 22g, protein 10g, fat 8g.

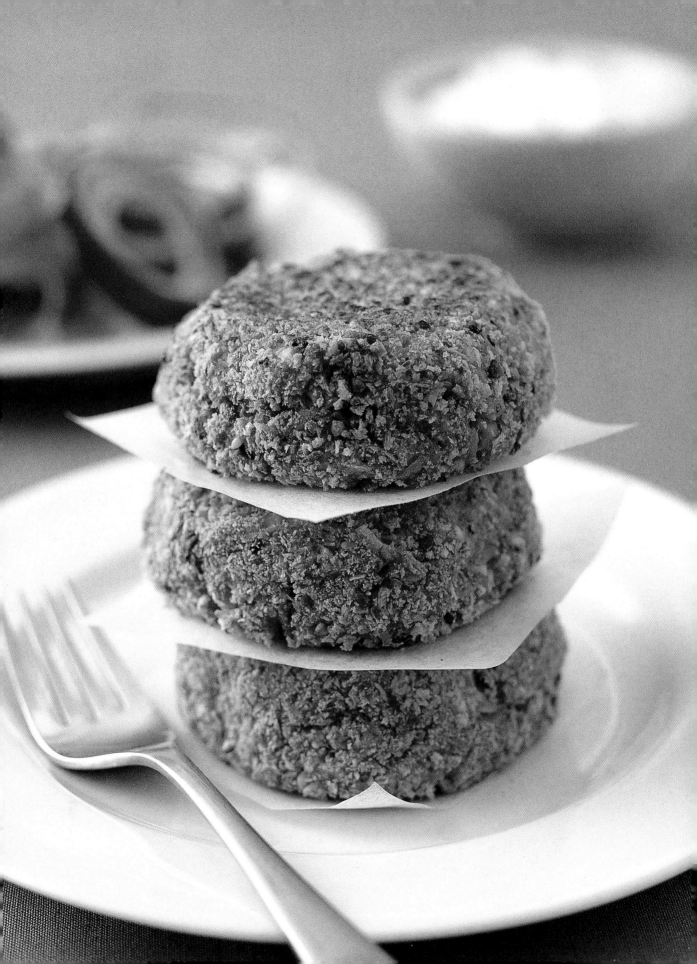

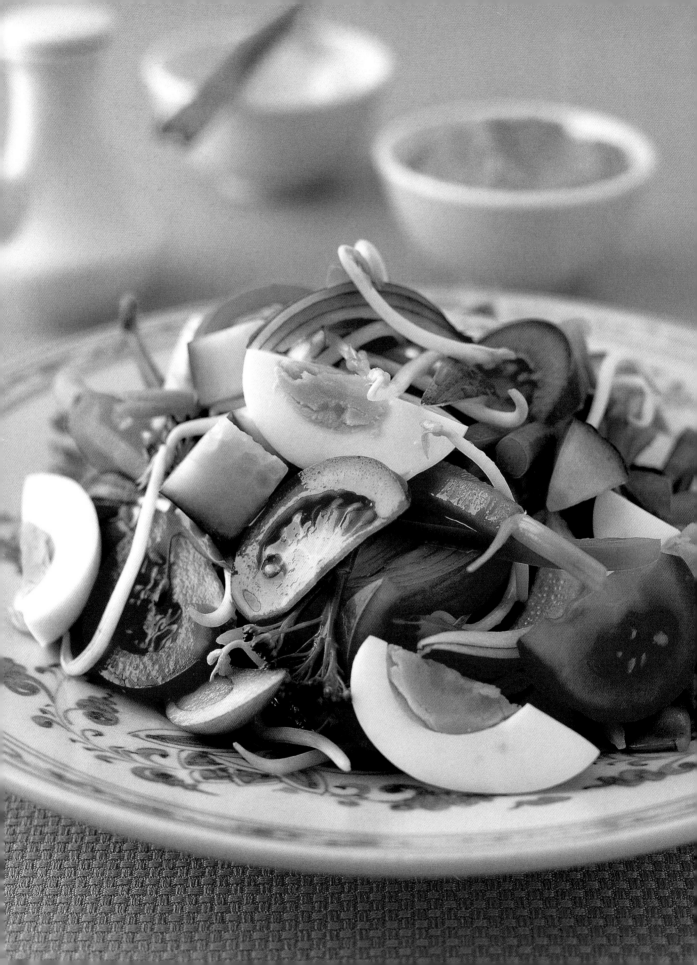

GADO GADO

- 1 cup (120g) bean shoots
- 1 cup (120g) green beans, string removed
- 1½ cups (110g) broccoli florets
- 1 cup (135g) carrot rings
- 1 cup (90g) cabbage, diced
- 1 medium green capsicum (bell pepper), diced
- 6–10 snow peas
- 2 tomatoes, cut into wedges
- 2 onions, cut into wedges
- 1 small cucumber, peeled and diced
- 2 hard-boiled eggs, cut into quarters

⏱ 30 minutes

VARIATION: Change vegetables according to season or taste.

METHOD

1. Half fill a medium saucepan with water and bring to a rapid boil.
2. Plunge the vegetables, except the tomatoes and cucumber, one variety at a time, into the boiling water for no more than one minute, or until the colour intensifies. Quickly remove the blanched vegetables from the water, place in the colander and immediately flush with cold, running water; this preserves the colour and crispness. Bring water back to the boil before blanching each type of vegetable. Alternatively, microwave vegetables with 2 tablespoons water on 'high' for two minutes.
3. Arrange all the ingredients on a platter. Serve as an appetizer or entrée at either room temperature or chilled with cooked brown rice and a dish of warm satay sauce (see recipe, page 163).

NUTRITION DATA PER SERVING:
103 kcal (433 kJ), CHO 10g, protein 9g, fat 3g.

CLAYTONS QUICHE

SERVES FOUR

- 4 eggs
- 1 cup (250ml) skimmed milk
- 1 cup (250g) wholemilk natural yoghurt
- 2 tablespoons wholemeal flour
- 1 cup (250g) ricotta cheese
- ½ cup (50g) chopped spring onions
- 120g mushrooms, sliced
- 1 medium tomato, diced
- oil
- 330g can asparagus, drained

⏱ 1 hour

This quiche makes its own crust. It is quick and easy to make, and is delicious hot or cold served with crusty bread and a green salad.

METHOD
1. Beat together eggs, milk, yoghurt and flour.
2. Add cheese, spring onions, mushrooms and tomato.
3. Pour into a lightly oiled flan dish.
4. Arrange asparagus on top.
5. Bake in a preheated 180°C (350°F) oven for 30–35 minutes or until quiche is set and lightly browned.

NUTRITION DATA PER SERVING:
274 kcal (1146 kJ), CHO 15g, protein 23g, fat 14g.

PITTA PIZZA

SERVES FOUR

- 4 small wholemeal pitta breads
- 1 cup tomato and basil sauce (see recipe, page 164) or 1 cup (250ml) commercial pasta sauce
- 3 large tomatoes, sliced
- 1 medium green capsicum (bell pepper), de-seeded and sliced
- 1 cup (70g) sliced mushrooms
- 1 medium onion, peeled and sliced
- 8 tablespoons grated, reduced-fat cheddar cheese
- oil
- 16 black olives, chopped (optional)
- 1 courgette, sliced (optional)

⏱ 30 minutes

The beauty of this recipe is that by using pitta bread as the pizza base, you can put the whole dish together very quickly making it an ideal snack or light meal. The pizzas also freeze well.

1. Spread pitta breads with sauce. Arrange the vegetables evenly over the top and sprinkle with grated cheese.
2. Place on a lightly oiled baking tray. Bake in a preheated 180°C (350°F) oven for 20 minutes or until cheese melts and begins to brown.
3. Serve pitta pizzas straight from the oven, accompanied by a tossed salad (see recipe, page 153).

NUTRITION DATA PER SERVING:
335 kcal (1404 kJ), CHO 42g, protein 17g, fat 11g.

SPANISH OMELETTE

SERVES FIVE

- 2 teaspoons margarine
- 3 medium potatoes, diced but not peeled
- 1 large onion, chopped
- 6 mushrooms, chopped
- 1 green capsicum (bell pepper), chopped
- ½ cup (70g) cooked vegetables (e.g. corn, peas, carrots)
- ½ stick celery, chopped
- 5 eggs
- ¼ teaspoon black pepper
- ¼ teaspoon ground nutmeg
- 1 teaspoon dried mixed herbs
- pinch salt (optional)
- 2 teaspoons chopped parsley
- few drops Tabasco sauce or pinch cayenne pepper
- ¼ (60ml) cup water

⏱ 45 minutes

Delicious cold or hot, this omlette is a great way of using up leftover cooked and uncooked vegetables. It also makes a nutritious school or office lunch.

METHOD

1. Melt margarine in frying pan over medium-high heat.
2. Add potato and onion. Cover and cook over low heat for approximately 15 minutes until potatoes are tender.
3. Add mushrooms, capsicum, cooked vegetables and celery and cook a further five minutes.
4. Beat eggs with seasonings and water.
5. Pour over vegetables in frying pan, cover, and cook over low heat until almost set. Do not allow bottom to burn.
6. Preheat grill to medium, and slide omelette under the grill to complete cooking.
7. Loosen omelette and turn onto warm plate.
8. Cut into wedges to serve.

NUTRITION DATA PER SERVING:
164 kcal (688 kJ), CHO 16g, protein 10g, fat 7g.

SPINACH FETTUCCINE

SERVES FOUR

This dish should always be eaten freshly prepared.

- ◆ 2 bunches fresh spinach or 500g frozen spinach
- ◆ 250g spinach fettuccine
- ◆ 2 tablespoons pine nuts
- ◆ 1 tablespoon water
- ◆ 1 small onion, finely chopped
- ◆ ½ clove garlic, crushed
- ◆ 1 teaspoon chopped fresh basil, or ½ teaspoon dried basil
- ◆ coarsely ground black pepper to taste
- ◆ 250g ricotta cheese

⏱ 30 minutes

METHOD

1. Trim away the roots and woody ends of the stems of fresh spinach.
2. Rinse spinach thoroughly in cold, running water, but do not dry. Heat a large saucepan. Put the spinach into the saucepan, cover and cook over medium-high heat for five to eight minutes or until tender. Remove from heat and drain in a colander. Set aside. If you are using frozen spinach, place it in a saucepan and thaw over low–medium heat. Remove from heat, drain well and squeeze to remove excess liquid. Set aside.
3. Fill a large saucepan two-thirds with water, and bring to a rapid boil. Add the fettuccine and boil for 10–12 minutes or until it is al dente (tender, but firm to the bite). Drain.
4. Meanwhile, in a dry frying pan, brown the pine nuts over medium heat, stirring constantly to ensure even colouring and to prevent burning. Remove from frying pan and set aside.
5. Return frying pan to the heat. Add the tablespoon of water, onion, garlic, basil and pepper. Cook over low heat until the onion is translucent.
6. In a large saucepan, combine the cooked spinach, pine nuts, ricotta cheese and the onion mixture. Add the fettuccine, use two forks to gently lift and turn mixture to combine well.
7. Serve hot.

NUTRITION DATA PER SERVING:
376 kcal (1573 kJ), CHO 47g, protein 20g, fat 11g.

SPINACH RAVIOLI WITH FRESH TOMATO SAUCE

SERVES FOUR

- 6 large ripe tomatoes, roughly chopped
- 1 teaspoon sugar
- 1 teaspoon chopped fresh basil or ½ teaspoon dried basil
- pinch tarragon
- 375g fresh spinach ravioli
- ½ cup (60g) grated reduced-fat cheddar cheese, or 2 tablespoons grated parmesan cheese

⏱ 45 minutes

METHOD

1. Place tomatoes, sugar and herbs in saucepan and simmer gently until mixture forms a thick sauce.
2. While tomatoes are cooking, three-quarter fill a second saucepan with cold water and rapidly bring to boil. Add ravioli and cook until tender. Drain.
3. Pour sauce over ravioli and mix gently.
4. Sprinkle with cheese.

NUTRITION DATA PER SERVING:

312 kcal (1307 kJ), CHO 51g, protein 15g, fat 5g.

POTATO GNOCCHI

SERVES FOUR

- 500g potatoes, peeled, cooked and mashed
- ½ cup (70g) plain flour
- ½ cup (70g) wholemeal flour
- 1 quantity fresh vegetable sauce (see recipe, page 164)
- 4 tablespoons grated, reduced-fat cheddar cheese

⏱ 15 minutes

VARIATION: Sprinkle with 4 tablespoons chopped lean ham, or use tomato and basil sauce (see recipe, page 164) instead of fresh vegetable sauce.

METHOD

1. Half fill saucepan with water and place on stove to boil. A little salt may be added to the cooking water if desired.
2. Mix potato with both flours, then turn onto a floured board and knead gently until smooth.
3. Divide mixture into four, and roll each into a sausage about 2cm in diameter. Cut lengths into 2cm pieces and drop into boiling water.
4. Boil gently for eight to ten minutes until gnocchi are light and cooked (gnocchi will rise to surface of the water as they cook).
5. Use a slotted spoon to remove onto a serving dish.
6. Toss in sauce, sprinkle with cheese and serve immediately.

NUTRITION DATA PER SERVING:

292 kcal (1222 kJ), CHO 50g, protein 14g, fat 4g.

SEMOLINA GNOCCHI WITH TOMATO AND BASIL SAUCE

SERVES FOUR

- 1½ cups (375ml) skimmed or semi-skimmed milk
- ½ teaspoon ground nutmeg
- 1 cup (160g) semolina
- 2 eggs
- small amount of plain flour
- 1 cup (250ml) of tomato and basil sauce (see recipe, page 164) or 1 cup (250ml) commercial tomato-based pasta sauce

⏱ 30 minutes

Gnocchi are best served fresh, but you can refrigerate them for up to three days and then reheat by dropping in boiling water. Alternatively, freeze the uncooked gnocchi and cook when you need to serve them.

METHOD

1. Place milk and nutmeg in medium saucepan and bring to boil. Remove from heat and quickly stir in semolina.
2. Return to heat and stir for one minute.
3. Add eggs and work into a smooth dough.
4. Break off small, even-sized pieces about the size of a walnut, roll into balls and toss in a little flour.
5. Half fill a large saucepan with water and bring to the boil.
6. Drop gnocchi into boiling water and cook for about five minutes (gnocchi will rise to the top of the water as they cook).
7. Drain. Toss in sauce and serve immediately.

NUTRITION DATA PER SERVING:
257 kcal (1076 kJ), CHO 38g, protein 12g, fat 6g.

BUBBLE AND SQUEAK

SERVES FOUR

- 2 teaspoons oil
- 1 medium onion, finely sliced
- 4 cups (600g) cooked, mixed vegetables (e.g. potato, cabbage, pumpkin, carrot, cauliflower, broccoli, beans, peas, spinach and courgette)
- black pepper to taste

⏱ 10 minutes

METHOD

1. In a frying pan, heat the oil. Add the onion and sauté gently until lightly browned.
2. Add mixed vegetables and pepper. Use a metal spatula to lift and turn mixture until well combined. Then press down vegetables to make a flat cake in the frying pan.
3. Cook over medium heat for five minutes, or until the bottom of the 'cake' is well browned.
4. Cut into wedges in the frying pan. Serve brown side up.

NUTRITION DATA PER SERVING:
106 kcal (445 kJ), CHO 13g, protein 7g, fat 3g.

SWEET POTATO AND BEAN RISOTTO

SERVES FOUR

- ◆ 2 cloves garlic, finely chopped
- ◆ 1 medium onion, peeled and sliced
- ◆ 2 teaspoons curry powder
- ◆ 4 cups (1 litre) vegetarian stock or 3 cups (750ml) stock and 1 cup (250ml) dry white wine
- ◆ 2 cups (410g) arborio rice, well washed
- ◆ 1 cup (140g) sweet potato, peeled and cut into 2.5cm cubes
- ◆ 1 cup (120g) green beans, prepared and cut into 4cm pieces
- ◆ black pepper, to taste
- ◆ 2 rounded tablespoons ricotta cheese
- ◆ 2 tablespoons grated parmesan cheese

🕐 20 minutes

The ingredients in a risotto can be greatly varied according to taste and available ingredients. Traditionally arborio rice is used but by using long grain, short grain or brown rice you can change the texture and flavour of the dish.

METHOD

1. In a large saucepan, sauté garlic, onion and curry powder in a little stock and set aside.
2. Wash rice well.
3. Place remainder of stock in saucepan and bring to boil.
4. Add ½ cup rice and gently stir until stock boils again. Repeat until all the rice is added to the pan.
5. Add the onions and sweet potato.
6. Reduce heat and cook gently, stirring occasionally, for around 10 minutes.
7. Add the beans and black pepper and cook for a further five minutes or until the rice is cooked and all stock absorbed.
8. Remove risotto from heat and stir in ricotta cheese.
9. Serve on individual plates and sprinkle with parmesan cheese.

NUTRITION DATA PER SERVING:
476 kcal (1996 kJ), CHO 83g, protein 24g, fat 5g.

VARIATION: MUSHROOM AND SUN-DRIED TOMATO
Replace sweet potato, green beans and curry powder with ½ cup (40g) sun-dried tomatoes, 1 cup (70g) sliced mushrooms and 1 cup (35g) baby spinach leaves. Add tomatoes and mushrooms early in the cooking process and toss the spinach through the mixture at the end of the cooking process.

VARIATION: CAPSICUM, BROCCOLI AND ASPARAGUS
Replace sweet potato, green beans and curry powder with ½ cup (60g) diced red capsicum (bell pepper), 1 cup (75g) broccoli florettes, ½ cup (70g) fresh asparagus pieces and 4 chopped spring onions. Add all vegetables early in cooking process.

VARIATION: PUMPKIN AND PEA
Replace sweet potato, green beans and curry powder with 1 cup (120g) diced pumpkin and 1 cup (160g) fresh or frozen peas. Add 2 tablespoons freshly chopped coriander or 1 teaspoon ground cumin to stock. Add pumpkin early in cooking process and peas later in the cooking process (note: fresh peas will require longer cooking than frozen ones).

BEAN CURD AND BEAN RED CURRY

SERVES FOUR

- ◆ 1 cup (120g) green beans
- ◆ 1 cup (70g) button mushrooms
- ◆ 400g firm tofu (soybean curd)
- ◆ 2 cups (500ml) semi-skimmed or skimmed evaporated milk
- ◆ 1 teaspoon coconut essence
- ◆ 1 tablespoon red curry paste
- ◆ 3 tablespoons fish sauce
- ◆ 2 teaspoons dark brown sugar
- ◆ 4 lime leaves
- ◆ 2 red chillies, de-seeded and sliced
- ◆ coriander leaves, for garnish

⏱ 10 minutes

METHOD

1. Top, tail and slice the green beans. Slice the mushrooms and cut the tofu into 2cm cubes.
2. Place milk, essence, curry paste, fish sauce, sugar and lime leaves in a wok or saucepan, stir and simmer for two minutes.
3. Add the mushrooms, green beans and tofu and simmer gently for another four to five minutes.
4. Remove lime leaves, stir in the sliced chillies.
5. Serve garnished with the coriander leaves.

NUTRITION DATA PER SERVING:
208 kcal (871 kJ), CHO 23g, protein 19g, fat 6g.

VEGETABLE CURRY

SERVES FOUR

- ◆ 500g mixed vegetables
- ◆ 2 teaspoons oil
- ◆ 1 onion, sliced
- ◆ 1 teaspoon ground turmeric
- ◆ ½ teaspoon ground cumin
- ◆ 2cm piece green ginger, chopped
- ◆ 2 cloves garlic, chopped
- ◆ 1 or 2 fresh hot chillies (optional), or chilli powder to taste
- ◆ 1 cup (250ml) water
- ◆ 1 cup (250ml) light coconut milk
- ◆ 1 tablespoon lemon juice

⏱ 45 minutes

Using a variety of vegetables makes this an economical dish based on vegetables in season. Beans, cabbage, broccoli, cauliflower, pumpkin, sweet potatoes, spinach, potatoes, peas, carrots, aubergine and courgette are ideal.

METHOD

1. Trim vegetables and cut into pieces.
2. Heat oil in wok or large frying pan until very hot .
3. Add onion and spices and toss until onion is golden brown.
4. Add the rest of the vegetables and stir-fry for two to three minutes.
5. Add water and cook for six to eight minutes, uncovered, or until vegetables are tender.
6. Add coconut milk and bring to boil.
7. Remove from heat. Add lemon juice.
8. Serve with brown rice.

NUTRITION DATA PER SERVING:
157 kcal (657 kJ), CHO 8g, protein 4g, fat 12g.

TOFU IN CHILLI SAUCE

SERVES FOUR

- 1 red capsicum (bell pepper), de-seeded and chopped
- 1 onion, peeled and sliced
- 1 cup (250ml) vegetable or chicken stock
- 2 cloves garlic, crushed or 1 teaspoon garlic paste
- 1 teaspoon finely chopped fresh ginger, or ginger paste
- 1 tablespoon sweet chilli sauce
- 2 tablespoons mirin (Japanese sweetened rice wine)
- 400g fresh soft tofu
- 2 spring onions, diagonally sliced
- 2 tablespoons chopped coriander

⏱ 10 minutes

METHOD
1. Simmer capsicum and onion in stock until soft.
2. Place in blender with garlic, ginger, chilli sauce and mirin and blend until smooth.
3. Bring to boil, reduce heat and simmer for two minutes.
4. Cut tofu into 2cm cubes, add to sauce and simmer gently for a further two minutes.
5. Use a slotted spoon to remove tofu; place on bed of cooked rice or noodles, pour over the sauce and sprinkle with spring onions and chopped coriander.

NUTRITION DATA PER SERVING:
80 kcal (337 kJ), CHO 2g, protein 8g, fat 6g.

TOFU SUKIYAKI

SERVES FOUR

- 3 cups (750ml) vegetable or meat stock
- 400g firm tofu, cut into 2cm cubes
- ¼ cup (60ml) mirin
- 1 tablespoon brown sugar
- 1 tablespoon citrus soy sauce
- 4 baby bok choy, cut into quarters
- 1 cup (135g) thinly sliced carrots
- 1 cup (120g) green beans, topped and tailed and diagonally sliced
- 1 cup (70g) mushrooms, thinly sliced
- 4 spring onions, sliced diagonally

⏱ 12 minutes

METHOD
1. Pour stock into wok and heat until just simmering.
2. Add tofu and simmer gently for one minute.
3. With a slotted spoon gently lift tofu from wok; set aside.
4. Add mirin, sugar and citrus soy to remaining stock in wok, stir to dissolve sugar and simmer for three minutes to reduce sauce.
5. Add bok choy, carrots, beans and mushrooms and cook for about two minutes or until they are just tender.
6. Add spring onions, return tofu to wok and gently combine with the other ingredients, being careful not to break up the tofu.
7. Serve with rice noodles or rice.

NUTRITION DATA PER SERVING:
112 kcal (469 kJ), CHO 10g, protein 9g, fat 6g.

CRÊPES AND PANCAKES

SERVES 4–5 (makes 12 large or 24 small
crêpes and 8–10 pancakes)

CRÊPES

- 1 cup (140g) wholemeal or plain
  white flour (or half-and-half)
- 3 eggs, lightly beaten
- 2 teaspoons oil or melted butter
- 1½ cups (375ml) skimmed milk

PANCAKES

- ¾ cup (100g) wholemeal or plain
  white flour (or half-and-half)
- 1 egg
- 1¼–1½ cups (300ml–375ml)
  skimmed milk

⏱ 1 hour 30 minutes

Crêpes are small, very thin pancakes; the raw batter is thinner than for traditional pancakes. Pancakes make a large, hearty wrapping for a variety of fillings. The cooked pancake should be about the size of a dinner plate and about 2mm thick. Both crêpes and pancakes are simple to make and very versatile. With either savoury or sweet fillings, use them for entrées, main courses, desserts or snacks. You will find that crêpes made entirely with wholemeal flour tend to be heavy A half-and-half combination makes a nutritious and tasty version.

METHOD

1. Sift flour into a bowl (if using wholemeal flour, add any wheat husks left in sieve to the sifted flour). Make a well in the flour. Slowly add the beaten eggs, stirring continually to draw the ingredients together and prevent lumps forming.
2. Mix oil or melted butter with milk. Slowly add to flour mixture, stirring continually, to form a thin, smooth pouring consistency like that of thin pouring cream. If too thick, add more milk, a little at a time, until you have the right consistency. (If you prefer, use a food processor or blender and simply add all the ingredients at once and process until smooth.)
3. Transfer batter to a jug and leave to stand in a cool place for at least an hour. If the mixture has thickened, add more milk, a little at a time, to the consistency of thin pouring cream.
4. Lightly grease a crêpe or heavy-bottomed frying pan and heat until very hot, but not smoking. Pour in 2–4 tablespoons of batter, depending on size of pan, and tilt pan to spread batter evenly.
5. When fine bubbles appear on the surface of the crêpe (or pancake) and it appears dry, use an egg slice or spatula to flip over and cook the other side for approximately five seconds until pale golden brown.
6. Repeat these steps for the remainder of the batter, brushing the pan with a little oil between crêpes and stacking them as they are cooked. Keep them covered with a damp tea-towel until you need them.

CRÊPES AND PANCAKES (continued)

7. Use any of the filling mixtures listed below, or create your own. Crêpes and pancakes can be filled and then served rolled up or folded in half or in quarters.

NUTRITION DATA PER SERVING OF CRÊPES (3 large crêpes):
231 kcal (968 kJ), CHO 29g, protein 12g, fat 7g.

NUTRITION DATA PER SERVING OF PANCAKES (2 pancakes):
186 kcal (778 kJ), CHO 26g, protein 9g, fat 5g.

SAVOURY FILLINGS FOR CRÊPES OR PANCAKES

Allow three large crêpes or two pancakes per serving. Fill pancakes with any of the fillings that follow, and top with low-fat natural yoghurt, ricotta cheese or a fine sprinkling of parmesan cheese. Serve the filled pancakes hot, accompanied by a crisp, green salad.

Asparagus
Cooked or canned asparagus spears or pieces tossed in cheese sauce (see recipe, page 163).

Mushroom and onion
Sliced mushrooms and onions cooked in a frying pan brushed with oil and tossed in white sauce (see recipe, page 162).

Ratatouille
Ratatouille sauce (see recipe, page 165) and topped with grated reduced-fat cheddar cheese.

Spinach
Cooked, chopped spinach mixed with ricotta cheese, sautéed spring onions, chopped basil and pine nuts.

Red kidney beans and corn

Sauté one medium finely diced capsicum (bell pepper) and one medium finely chopped onion in 3 tablespoons water for approximately three minutes until soft. Add 1 cup drained canned red kidney beans, 1 cup drained canned corn kernels, 2 tablespoons tomato purée, ½ teaspoon ground oregano and a small pinch chilli powder. Simmer gently for five to ten minutes until the liquid is almost evaporated. Fill the pancakes and roll them up. Sprinkle with 4 tablespoons low-fat grated cheese, and grill to melt the cheese topping.

Meat-based fillings

Seafood

500g seafood (e.g. marinara mix) cooked in one quantity of tomato and basil sauce (see recipe, page 164).

Chicken and avocado

Two sliced cooked chicken fillets and one sliced avocado tossed in one quantity of cheese sauce (see recipe, page 163).

Savoury beef

500g lean minced beef cooked in one quantity of tomato and basil sauce (see recipe, page 164). Fill crêpes or pancakes and top with low-fat natural yoghurt or ricotta cheese, or a fine sprinkling of parmesan cheese.

Steak and onion

Slice 500g fillet steak into very thin strips, and marinate in 2 tablespoons Worcestershire sauce and 1 crushed clove of garlic for 10 minutes. Sauté beef in 2 teaspoons oil for three minutes. Add one large sliced onion and sauté for another two minutes. Add ¼ cup (60ml) red wine, and simmer for one to two minutes. Thicken with 1 tablespoon cornflour blended with 2 tablespoons water. Fill pancakes and serve them topped with low-fat natural yoghurt and a sprinkling of chopped parsley.

VEGETABLE SIDE DISHES

Vegetables have tended to become a neglected part of the meal. Yet, with a little imagination, they can be a real feature. Try mixing vegetables in different combinations, and experiment with adding fresh or dried herbs and seasonings. Nutmeg, curry powder, onion, chives, tomato, garlic, wine or a sprinkle of toasted sesame seeds or almonds provide a delicious flavour boost.

The following ideas may help get you started on a new appreciation of the versatility of vegetables. All the suggestions are for four people.

Braised onion

Place 1 cup (250ml) water and 1 chicken stock cube in a saucepan and bring to the boil. Add 4 small peeled and sliced onions and simmer them for about eight minutes until tender. Lift out the onions and set them aside, add 2 tablespoons dry white wine to the stock and boil the liquid until it is reduced to about 3 tablespoons. Add the onions, heat through and serve them garnished with chopped chives or parsley.

Braised lettuce

Wash an Iceberg lettuce and remove any stalks or damaged outside leaves. Cut the lettuce into wedges. Bring 2 cups (500ml) chicken stock to the boil, drop in the lettuce wedges and simmer them for 15–20 seconds. Lift them out and, if desired, serve them garnished with finely sliced spring onion tops.

Lemon broccoli

Wash 1 large head of broccoli, removing the woody stem. Cut the broccoli into even florets and steam or boil them for four to six minutes until they are tender but still crisp. Drain the broccoli.

Alternatively, microwave on high for four minutes. Finally, toss in a mixture of lemon juice, the rind of 1 lemon and 2 teaspoons toasted sesame seeds.

Spinach and spring onions

Wash a bunch of fresh spinach under running water, remove all trace of dirt and the woody stems. Chop the spinach finely and place it in a saucepan with a bunch of chopped spring onions, 2 tablespoons finely chopped parsley, a pinch of nutmeg and 2 tablespoons water. Cover and cook for five to six minutes. Alternatively, cover and microwave it on high for four to five minutes. Serve immediately.

Diced parsleyed potatoes

Scrub 4 medium potatoes and cut them into 2cm cubes. Drop into boiling water and simmer gently for 8–10 minutes until tender. Drain. Alternatively, microwave on high for seven to eight minutes. Finally, sprinkle them with parsley and toss gently.

Snow peas and asparagus

Cut 20 asparagus spears to about the length of the snow peas, discarding the woody ends. Plunge the asparagus into boiling water for two minutes until the asparagus spears are tender. Add twenty snow peas, return to the boil and then drain. Make sure that the vegetables don't overcook. Place them on a serving dish and sprinkle them with toasted sesame seeds or almond slivers. This recipe can be varied by replacing the asparagus with whole green beans or celery strips, microwaved on high for two to three minutes.

Succotash (peas, capsicum and corn)

Boil or steam 1–1½ cups (160–240g) each of frozen peas and corn kernels for four to five minutes. Drain. Alternatively, cover and microwave on high for four minutes. Then add a diced red capsicum (bell pepper), mix thoroughly, season with freshly ground black pepper and serve.

Pumpkin and mushrooms

Peel and seed 4 medium pieces of pumpkin and slice each into pieces about 1cm thick. Place them in a saucepan with 6 sliced mushrooms, 1 cup (250ml) unsweetened tomato juice, 1 crushed clove garlic and ground black pepper. Simmer gently for about 15 minutes until the vegetables are tender or, alternatively, place all the ingredients in a microwave dish, cover and microwave on high for eight minutes.

Courgette and carrot rings

Trim and thickly slice 4 medium courgettes and cut ½ medium carrot into thin rings. Heat 2 teaspoons oil in a large saucepan, add the carrots and cook, tossing them constantly, for two minutes. Add the courgettes and cook, tossing them constantly, for a further two minutes. Add ½ cup (125ml) water, cover and cook for about five minutes until tender. Drain and season with ground black pepper and chopped parsley.

Leek and apple

Wash and slice a large leek. Peel and slice a large cooking apple. Heat a tablespoon of water in a saucepan, add the leek and apple and toss them to mix. Cover and cook over low heat for approximately eight minutes until tender. Alternatively, microwave the leek, apple and water on high for five minutes.

Courgette creole

Peel and quarter 1 medium onion, cut ½ medium green capsicum (bell pepper) into strips. Place in a saucepan with 2 tablespoons of water and cook for two minutes. Add 4 quartered tomatoes, 4 courgettes cut into wedges, 12 pitted black olives and ½ teaspoon of chopped fresh basil (or ¼ teaspoon dried basil), cover and simmer gently for 10 minutes.

WILD RICE PILAF

SERVES FOUR TO SIX

- 1 cup (200g) long grain and wild rice mix
- 2 teaspoons vegetable oil
- 1 small onion, finely diced
- 4 mushrooms, cut into small dice
- 1 red capsicum (bell pepper), cut into small dice
- ½ green capsicum (bell pepper), cut into small dice
- 2 stalks celery, cut into small dice
- ¼ cup (30g) slivered almonds, toasted until lightly browned
- ¼ cup (30g) pecans, chopped
- 2 tablespoons fresh parsley, chopped
- pepper and salt
- 8–10 drops Tabasco sauce
- 1 teaspoon Worcestershire sauce

🕐 50 minutes

METHOD

1. Bring 3–4 cups water to a boil in a large saucepan. Add the rice, return to the boil, then turn down and simmer until the rice is tender (about 15 minutes). Drain and set aside.
2. Heat the oil in a large frying pan, then add the onion and mushrooms and sauté until the onion is clear. Add the other vegetables and cook for a further three to four minutes, or until the vegetables are just cooked but still retain some crunch.
3. Add the rice to the vegetable mixture with the almonds, pecans and parsley.
4. Flavour with the pepper and salt, Tabasco and Worcestershire sauces and toss well to thoroughly combine the flavours.
5. Serve on a warm plate with an accompaniment such as cajun fish (see recipe page 79), garnished with a wedge of lemon or lime.

NUTRITION DATA PER SERVING:
253 kcal (1060 kJ), CHO 29g, protein 6g, fat 12g.

COUSCOUS

SERVES SIX

- 2 cups (250ml) water
- 2 cups (380g) couscous

🕐 5 minutes

VARIATION: To increase the flavour, use stock to replace water when cooking. After couscous swells stir in two finely chopped spring onions and/or finely chopped cooked mushrooms.

One of the good things about couscous is the speed with which it can be prepared.

METHOD

1. Place water in a large saucepan and bring to the boil.
2. Remove from heat and stir in couscous.
3. Cover and stand for two to three minutes to allow it to swell.
4. Place back over heat for a further two to three minutes, stirring with a fork to separate the grains.

NUTRITION DATA PER SERVING:
221 kcal (925 kJ), CHO 38g, protein 7g, fat 1g.

COURGETTE AND TOMATO BAKE

SERVES FOUR

- ◆ 2 teaspoons margarine or oil
- ◆ 1 round of lavash bread
- ◆ 2 medium courgettes,
  cut in half crossways, and then
  into strips
- ◆ 3 tomatoes, sliced
- ◆ 4 spring onions, chopped
- ◆ 2 teaspoons fresh herbs, chopped,
  or 1 teaspoon dried mixed herbs
- ◆ pinch salt (optional)
- ◆ pinch pepper
- ◆ ½ medium onion, sliced
- ◆ 1 tablespoon tahini
- ◆ juice of ½ lemon
- ◆ ¼ teaspoon finely chopped or
  minced fresh ginger
- ◆ ¼ teaspoon prepared mustard
- ◆ 2 tablespoons sesame seeds

⏱ 15 minutes

METHOD

1. Spread margarine or oil over casserole.
2. Place bread in casserole. Push into corners without breaking it, and leave excess hanging out.
3. Place half of the courgettes in the bottom.
4. Cover with the sliced tomato.
5. Sprinkle spring onions, herbs, salt and pepper over.
6. Add the remainder of the courgettes over, then the finely sliced onion.
7. Blend tahini, lemon juice, ginger, mustard and a little water to make a thin paste and pour over vegetables.
8. Sprinkle with sesame seeds.
9. Fold edges of bread in around the edge of the casserole to form a crust around the edge.
10. Bake in a preheated 200°C (400°F) oven for 40–45 minutes or until the bread is brown and crusty, and the courgettes are tender.

NUTRITION DATA PER SERVING:
151 kcal (633 kJ), CHO 21g, protein 7g, fat 4g.

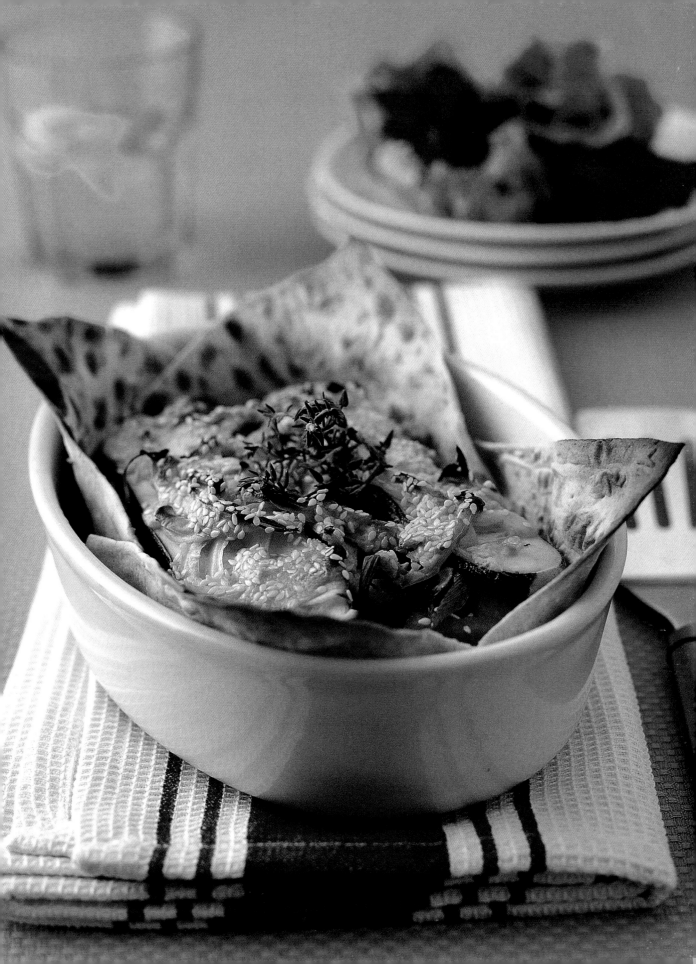

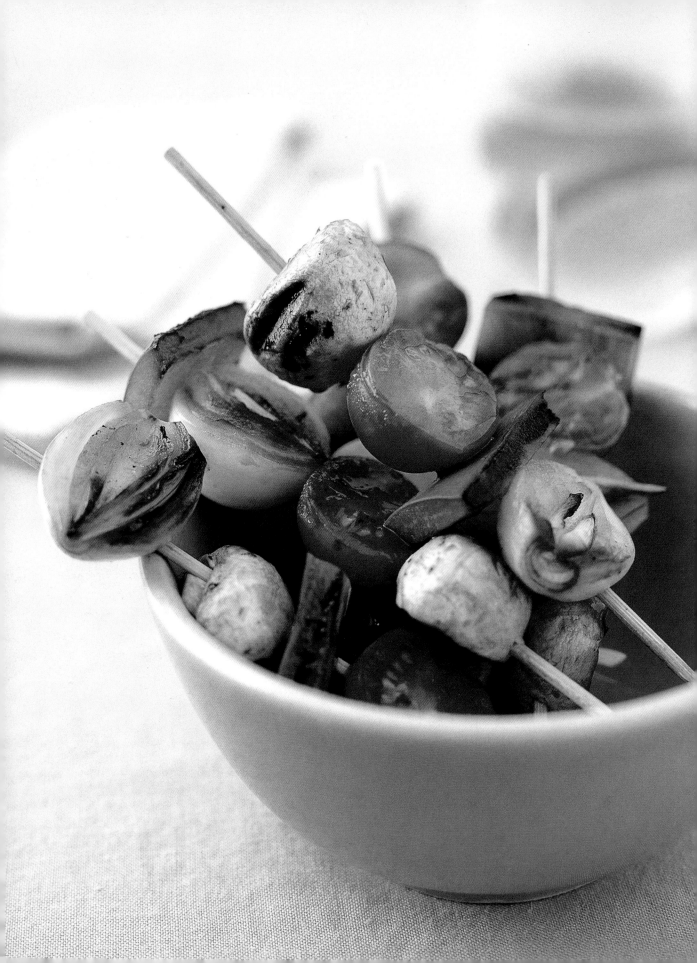

VEGETABLES EN BROCHETTE

SERVES FOUR

- 16 cherry tomatoes
- 16 pearl onions, peeled (or small pieces of onion)
- 16 button mushrooms, stalks trimmed
- 1 medium green capsicum (bell pepper), cut into 2cm squares
- 2 tablespoons lemon juice
- 2 teaspoons soy sauce

⏱ 20 minutes

Serve these with rice or on a bed of cracked wheat and you have the basis of a delectable meal.

METHOD

1. Thread vegetables evenly along eight 18cm skewers, leaving about 2.5cm of skewer free at each end.
2. Mix lemon juice and soy sauce, and brush mixture over vegetables.
3. Grill for about five minutes on each side until vegetables are tender. During grilling, brush with lemon juice and soy sauce mixture at intervals to prevent drying.
4. Serve hot.

NUTRITION DATA PER SERVING:
33 kcal (139 kJ), CHO 5g, protein 3g, fat trace.

ORANGE-GLAZED PARSNIPS

SERVES FOUR

- 2 medium parsnips, scrubbed and sliced
- 1 teaspoon grated orange rind
- ½ cup (125ml) orange juice
- 2 teaspoons margarine

⏱ 15 minutes

VARIATION: Carrots cooked this way are splendid, too.

METHOD

1. Drop parsnips into boiling water and cook until almost tender (about five minutes), or microwave, covered, with 2 tablespoons of water for three minutes until almost tender.
2. Drain and add orange rind, juice and margarine.
3. Bring to boil and cook for a further three minutes, or microwave, covered, on high for a further two minutes.
4. Lift out parsnips and keep warm.
5. Return saucepan to heat and simmer orange sauce to allow it to reduce and thicken.
6. Once sauce has thickened pour over parsnips, reheat quickly and serve.

NUTRITION DATA PER SERVING:
59 kcal (246 kJ), CHO 8g, protein 1g, fat 2g.

DRY CURRY OF POTATO, AUBERGINE AND PEA

SERVES FOUR

- 1 tablespoon ghee or unsalted butter or margarine
- 1½ teaspoon panch phora (Indian five spices)
- 1 large onion, finely chopped
- 2 tablespoons chopped mint
- 1 teaspoon finely chopped fresh ginger
- ¼ teaspoon ground chilli
- 1 teaspoon ground turmeric
- 500g potatoes, peeled and diced
- 500g aubergine, diced
- 250g frozen or fresh green peas
- 3 tablespoons hot water
- 1 teaspoon garam masala
- 1 tablespoon lemon juice
- salt to taste (optional)

⏱ 45 minutes

Spices used in Indian curries are usually available in large supermarkets and are also readily available in Asian grocery shops. Panch phora is a mixture of five different types of seed used whole—one part fenugreek seeds and fennel seeds to two parts black mustard seeds, cumin seeds and black cumin seeds. Garam masala is a mixture of ground spices which may vary in type and amount, e.g. coriander, cumin, cardamom, cinnamon, cloves and nutmeg. Both panch phora and garam masala can be purchased pre-mixed.

METHOD

1. Heat the ghee and fry the panch phora until seeds start to brown.
2. Add onion and fry until soft.
3. Add mint, ginger, chilli and turmeric and stir.
4. Add vegetables and water, mix well and cover.
5. Reduce to a low heat and cook for 20 minutes shaking pan occasionally to toss vegetables and to prevent them burning.
6. Sprinkle with garam masala, lemon juice and salt, cover and cook for a further 10 minutes.
7. Serve hot, accompanied by Indian lamb in spinach sauce (see recipe, page 104).

NUTRITION DATA PER SERVING:
175 kcal (734 kJ), CHO 24g, protein 8g, fat 5g.

SWEET POTATO PATTIES

SERVES FOUR

- 500g orange sweet potatoes
- ¼ teaspoon ground cardamom
- white pepper to taste
- ¼ teaspoon ground turmeric
- ½ teaspoon finely chopped or minced fresh ginger
- 2 teaspoons chopped parsley
- 2 tablespoons chopped chives
- ⅓ cup (50g) sesame seeds

⏱ 2 hours

VARIATION: Replace sesame seeds with wheatgerm.

METHOD

1. Peel sweet potatoes and cut into pieces.
2. Place in saucepan with 1–2 cups (250ml–500ml) water and the cardamom, and cook until tender. Alternatively, steam or microwave the sweet potato.
3. Drain, remove the cardamom and mash the potatoes. Add the other spices, ginger, parsley and chives. Then cover and cool (approximately 1 hour).
4. Shape into patties (four large or eight small) and coat with sesame seeds.
5. Place on baking tray. Bake in a preheated 200°C (400°F) oven for approximately 30 minutes or until sesame seeds are toasted and patties are heated through.

NUTRITION DATA PER SERVING:
167 kcal (699 kJ), CHO 29g, protein 7g, fat 2g.

MUSHROOM AND PECAN RICE

SERVES FOUR

- ½ cup chicken stock (see recipe, page 68) or 1 stock cube in ½ cup (125ml) water
- 6 mushrooms, sliced
- 4 spring onions, cut into 1cm lengths
- 2 tablespoons chopped pecan nuts
- 2 cups (380g) cooked brown or basmati rice

⏱ 15 minutes

This filling dish is wonderfully quick to prepare. Try using walnuts or pine nuts instead of pecan nuts. If you decide to use onions in place of the spring onions, then add a tablespoon of chopped parsley as well.

METHOD

1. Heat chicken stock in large pan or wok.
2. Cook mushrooms and onions in stock for three to four minutes.
3. Add nuts and rice and toss while heating through. Serve hot or chill and serve cold.

NUTRITION DATA PER SERVING:
183 kcal (767 kJ), CHO 31g, protein 4g, fat 5g.

MUSHROOM STROGANOFF

SERVES FOUR

- ◆ 2 tablespoons water
- ◆ 2 onions, sliced
- ◆ 1 red or green capsicum (bell pepper), diced
- ◆ 16–20 medium-sized button mushrooms, sliced
- ◆ 3 spring onions, chopped
- ◆ 2 teaspoons paprika
- ◆ 1 cup (250g) low-fat, natural yoghurt
- ◆ 3 tablespoons chopped parsley

⏱ 15 minutes

Serve this dish with basmati rice, noodles or beancurd, or use it as a topping for jacket potatoes. It makes an excellent piquant sauce for grilled meats or fillets of chicken and fish.

METHOD

1. In the frying pan, bring the water to a simmer and add the onion, red or green capsicum and the mushrooms. Simmer gently for five minutes.
2. Add spring onions and paprika and simmer gently, stirring occasionally, for a further five minutes, or microwave for a further two minutes on high. Remove from heat.
3. Place yoghurt in a bowl, gradually fold in mushroom mixture. Do not reheat as yoghurt will curdle. Garnish.

NUTRITION DATA PER SERVING:
59 kcal (249 kJ), CHO 8g, protein 6g, fat 1g.

CURRIED POTATOES AND CAULIFLOWER

SERVES FOUR

- ◆ 1–2 teaspoons curry powder (according to taste)
- ◆ 2 medium potatoes, scrubbed and diced
- ◆ ½ cauliflower, separated into florets
- ◆ 1 bay leaf
- ◆ 1 cup (250ml) boiling water
- ◆ 2 teaspoons chopped parsley

⏱ 30 minutes

The flavour of curried food improves with standing, so this dish can be prepared 24 hours in advance and stored, well covered, in the refrigerator. Reheat before serving.

METHOD

1. Dry fry the curry powder in the base of large saucepan for one minute, stirring constantly.
2. Add all the other ingredients except the parsley.
3. Cover saucepan and leave to simmer gently for 20 minutes, or until vegetables are tender and the water absorbed. Remove bay leaf. Serve hot, garnished with parsley.

NUTRITION DATA PER SERVING:
52 kcal (218 kJ), CHO 9g, protein 3g, fat trace.

VEGETABLES JULIENNE

SERVES FOUR

- 1 small courgette
- 2 medium carrots
- 8 French beans
- 1 stick celery
- ½ green capsicum (bell pepper)
- 4 spring onions
- 1½ cups (375ml) water
- 1 chicken stock cube

⏱ 20 minutes

Prepare the vegetables neatly using a small sharp knife. Cook quickly and serve immediately.

METHOD

1. Trim top from courgette. Cut in half, across, then in half lengthways and, finally, into julienne strips.
2. Peel carrots, cut as for courgette. Top and tail beans. Cut each in half, across, then in half lengthways.
3. Cut celery into lengths, then into strips. Cut capsicum into strips, removing any pith and seeds.
4. Trim spring onions, cut into lengths, then each length in half.
5. Add water and stock cube to saucepan, bring to boil.
6. Add carrots and cook for two to three minutes, then beans, celery and courgette and cook a further minute.
7. Lastly, add capsicum and spring onions and cook for a further minute.
8. Drain, then gently lift vegetables from water, using tongs or a slotted spoon to avoid breaking strips.

NUTRITION DATA PER SERVING:
35 kcal (146 kJ), CHO 6g, protein 2g, fat trace.

HOT SHREDDED BEETS

SERVES FOUR

- 2 medium beetroot
- 2 teaspoons margarine
- 6 spring onions, chopped
- ¼ teaspoon black pepper
- pinch salt (optional)

⏱ 20 minutes

Beetroot has a piquancy that adds contrast to a meal.

METHOD

1. Top and tail beets, peel and grate.
2. Heat margarine in a frying pan over medium–high heat, and add beetroot, spring onions, black pepper and salt.
3. Sauté gently, turning from time to time, for about 10 minutes or until cooked through.

NUTRITION DATA PER SERVING:
53 kcal (222 kJ), CHO 7g, protein 2g, fat 2g.

SPICED RICE WITH PEAS

SERVES FOUR

- ◆ 1 tablespoon polyunsaturated vegetable oil
- ◆ 1 teaspoon finely chopped fresh ginger
- ◆ ½ fresh chilli, finely chopped, or ½ teaspoon minced chilli paste
- ◆ ¼ teaspoon black mustard seeds
- ◆ ¼ teaspoon cumin seeds
- ◆ 3 cups (750ml) water
- ◆ 2 curry leaves
- ◆ 1 cup (200g) basmati rice
- ◆ 100g frozen peas
- ◆ 2 teaspoons each of fresh coriander, mint, and basil, chopped
- ◆ ¼ teaspoon ground saffron
- ◆ salt to taste

⏱ 25 minutes

METHOD

1. Heat oil in pan, add ginger, chilli, mustard and cumin seeds and cook, stirring, for one minute.
2. Add water, bring to boil and add all other ingredients, cover and return to boil.
3. Reduce heat and simmer for 15 minutes or until rice is tender.
4. Serve accompanied with mogul lamb (see recipe, page 105).

NUTRITION DATA PER SERVING:
235 kcal (985 kJ), CHO 42g, protein 5g, fat 5g.

AUBERGINE NEAPOLITAN

SERVES FOUR

- ◆ 1 large or 2 small aubergines, peeled and thinly sliced
- ◆ 4 large tomatoes, sliced
- ◆ 2 onions, sliced
- ◆ ½ teaspoon mixed dried herbs
- ◆ ground black pepper to taste
- ◆ 1 clove garlic, crushed
- ◆ 1 cup (250ml) tomato juice or purée

⏱ 1 hour

METHOD

1. Layer vegetables in casserole.
2. Sprinkle with herbs, pepper and garlic and pour over the tomato juice or purée.
3. Bake in a preheated 180°C (350°F) oven, uncovered, for 45 minutes.

NUTRITION DATA PER SERVING:
62 kcal (258 kJ), CHO 11g, protein 4g, fat trace.

CRACKED WHEAT

SERVES FOUR

- ½ cups (90g) burghul (cracked wheat)
- 1½ cups (375ml) chicken stock (see recipe, page 68)

⏱ 15 minutes

Carbohydrates should be central to meals. Cracked wheat prepared this way is a quick and easy way to build a meal, just as you would with rice or pasta.

METHOD

1. Wash wheat under cold running water.
2. Place in saucepan and pour chicken stock over. Simmer for 10–15 minutes until tender.

NUTRITION DATA PER SERVING:
139 kcal (593 kJ), CHO 26g, protein 6g, fat 1g.

ROAST WINTER VEGETABLE MEDLEY

SERVES FOUR

- 2 tablespoons olive oil
- 1 small swede, peeled
- 1 beetroot, peeled
- 1 potato, peeled
- 1 parsnip, peeled
- 1 onion, peeled
- 1 small sweet potato, peeled
- ½ small celeriac root (optional)
- freshly ground black pepper
- salt
- 1 tablespoon chopped fresh rosemary

⏱ 1 hour 15 minutes

METHOD

1. Preheat the oven to 200°C.
2. Place the oil in a baking dish and heat in the oven for five minutes.
3. Cut the swede, beetroot and potato into four pieces and steam or microwave until just beginning to soften.
4. Meanwhile, cut the celeriac, parsnip, onion and sweet potato into four pieces.
5. Remove the baking dish from the oven and place the vegetables in the hot oil, turning each piece so it is coated with oil.
6. Grind fresh pepper over the vegetables, sprinkle lightly with salt if desired and sprinkle the rosemary over.
7. Bake until the vegetables are tender and browned, about 45–60 minutes. Turn the vegetables at least once during the cooking period.

NUTRITION DATA PER SERVING:
172 kcal (720 kJ), CHO 18g, protein 4g, fat 10g.

VEGEBALLS

SERVES FOUR

- 2 teaspoons margarine
- 12 small white or pearl onions
- 12 button mushrooms (or canned champignons)
- 12 cherry tomatoes
- coarsely ground black pepper

🕐 15 minutes

VARIATION: Substitute small white or pearl onions with 2cm lengths of spring onion.

METHOD
1. Melt margarine in pan or wok.
2. Add onions and toss gently for three to four minutes until beginning to soften.
3. Add mushrooms and continue tossing until they darken evenly.
4. Add tomatoes and very gently toss until they are heated through.
5. Sprinkle with black pepper.

NUTRITION DATA PER SERVING:
37 kcal (155 kJ), CHO 3g, protein 2g, fat 2g.

STIR-FRIED VEGETABLES

SERVES FOUR

- ½ Chinese cabbage or ⅛ green cabbage
- 1 teaspoon oil
- 1 teaspoon minced fresh ginger
- 1 small white onion, quartered
- ¾ cup (70g) broccoli florets
- 1 small carrot, finely sliced
- 10–12 snow peas
- ¾ cup (70g) bean shoots
- ½ green capsicum (bell pepper), diced
- 100g mushrooms, sliced
- ½ cup (125ml) water
- 1 stock cube
- 1 tablespoon soy sauce

🕐 20 minutes

Stir-fried vegetables should be crisp and brightly coloured—the result of swift cooking over high heat.

METHOD
1. Prepare the Chinese cabbage by cutting off the woody ends of stalks. Discard. Cut the stalks into 2cm lengths and shred the leaves. Cut the cabbage leaves into shreds about 5cm long.
2. Place wok or heavy frying pan over high heat. Coat thinly with the oil. When very hot add fresh ginger and onion. Stir-fry for two to three minutes.
3. Add remaining vegetables, stir-fry for two to three minutes more.
4. Dissolve the stock cube in water, then add to vegetables.
5. Turn the heat down, add the soy sauce and combine with the vegetables. Cover the wok or pan, and simmer vegetables for three to four minutes. Serve hot.

NUTRITION DATA PER SERVING:
41 kcal (172 kJ), CHO 6g, protein 4g, fat 1g.

SWEET AND SOUR RED CABBAGE

SERVES FOUR

- ◆ 500g red cabbage, shredded
- ◆ 1 onion, chopped
- ◆ 1 cooking apple, peeled, cored and chopped
- ◆ 1 clove garlic, crushed
- ◆ 1 tablespoon vinegar
- ◆ 1 teaspoon caraway seeds
- ◆ pepper to taste
- ◆ 3 tablespoons water

⏱ 30 minutes

This makes a good companion dish to rice, noodles or potato. Add a small portion of grilled fish or meat and you have a delicious, well-balanced meal.

METHOD

1. Place cabbage, onion, apple, garlic, vinegar, caraway seeds, and pepper in a saucepan or microwave-proof bowl.
2. Cook over a low heat for five minutes, stirring frequently or microwave on high for three minutes.
3. Add the water, bring to the boil and simmer for 10 minutes or microwave on high for a further five minutes.
4. Serve by arranging the cabbage on a hot serving dish, sprinkled with parsley.

NUTRITION DATA PER SERVING:
49 kcal (204 kJ), CHO 8g, protein 3g, fat trace.

CRUNCHY PEASANT RICE

SERVES FOUR

- ◆ ½ bunch spinach or silverbeet
- ◆ 1 tablespoon water
- ◆ 1 small onion, chopped
- ◆ 2 cups (380g) cooked brown or basmati rice
- ◆ 3 teaspoons soy sauce
- ◆ 2 tablespoons chopped brazil nuts

⏱ 10 minutes

VARIATION: Almonds or pine nuts are as good in this dish as the brazil nuts.

METHOD

1. Wash spinach or silverbeet thoroughly, and cook without any additional water in the saucepan, or microwave, for about two minutes.
2. Drain well and chop coarsely.
3. Heat large pan, add water and sauté onion until transparent.
4. Toss all ingredients lightly together in pan until heated through.

NUTRITION DATA PER SERVING:
226 kcal (945 kJ), CHO 37g, protein 6g, fat 6g.

SCALLOPED POTATOES

- 6 medium potatoes, scrubbed
- 1 cup (250ml) skimmed milk
- ¼ teaspoon coarsely ground black pepper
- 1 teaspoon chopped parsley
- ¼ teaspoon dried mixed herbs

⏱ 35 minutes

VARIATION: Omit the mixed herbs and sprinkle with sweet paprika to taste, or after the potatoes have been in the oven for 25 minutes, remove and sprinkle with grated, reduced-fat cheddar cheese, and then return to the oven for five minutes or until the topping is golden and bubbling.

This is wonderfully satisfying as it is, but lends itself equally to tempting variations. We have given two options, but you can experiment with your own. Although scalloped potatoes are usually eaten hot, they can also be served cold.

METHOD
1. Slice potatoes finely. Arrange in overlapping rows or circles in a shallow baking dish.
2. Pour over the skimmed milk and sprinkle with pepper, parsley and herbs.
3. Bake in a preheated 180°C (350°F) oven for 30 minutes or until potatoes are tender and slightly browned on top, or microwave, covered, on high for 20 minutes.
4. Serve hot with meat, fish or chicken.

NUTRITION DATA PER SERVING:
135 kcal (566 kJ), CHO 26g, protein 7g, fat trace.

JACKET POTATOES

SERVES FOUR AS AN ACCOMPANIMENT
OR TWO AS A LIGHT MEAL

♦ 4 medium-sized potatoes

⏱ 70 minutes

METHOD

1. Wash potatoes well, do not peel. Prick several times with a fork or skewer. For a crispy skin do not cover. For a softer skin wrap potatoes in foil.
2. Bake the potatoes in a preheated 180°C (350°F) oven for 45–60 minutes or until tender when tested with a skewer. Alternatively, cook uncovered in the microwave on high for 12 minutes, turning them over halfway through cooking.
3. Serve plain or try some of the following delicious fillings, or a combination of your own.

Cheese and pastrami

Slice tops off potatoes and scoop out flesh, leaving four firm shells. Cut two small, thin slices of pastrami into fine strips and mix with ½ cup (60g) grated reduced-fat cheddar cheese, the flesh from potatoes and 2 tablespoons low-fat milk. Add a little ground black pepper, spoon back into potato shells and reheat in oven for about five to ten minutes.

Cottage cheese (or yoghurt) and chives

Split open tops of potatoes and place ½ tablespoon cottage cheese or low-fat yoghurt in each. Sprinkle with chopped chives and serve immediately.

Tomato and onion

Sauté one finely chopped onion in a little water, add one medium chopped tomato, ½ teaspoon chopped fresh basil or oregano and a pinch of ground black pepper. Mix with flesh from potatoes, spoon into potato shells and reheat in oven for about five to ten minutes.

Spicy yoghurt

Combine the flesh of potatoes with 2 tablespoons low-fat natural yoghurt and a pinch each of ground ginger, cinnamon and cloves. Spoon back into potato shells and reheat in oven for about five to ten minutes.

DUCHESS POTATOES

SERVES FOUR

- 4 medium-sized old potatoes
- 1 egg
- 1 teaspoon margarine
- white pepper to taste
- pinch salt (optional)
- nutmeg

⏱ 30–40 minutes

METHOD

1. Wash, peel and rinse potatoes.
2. Cut into even-sized pieces.
3. Place in small quantity of boiling water and cook until soft (about 20 minutes) or microwave, covered, on high until soft.
4. Drain and mash potatoes.
5. Beat egg and put aside 1 teaspoon for glazing.
6. Beat potatoes, margarine and egg together until fluffy.
7. Season with pepper (and salt, if desired).
8. Pipe onto an oven tray to form cone shapes.
9. Glaze with remaining egg.
10. Sprinkle with nutmeg.
11. Brown in a preheated 200°C (400°F) oven for 10 minutes.

NUTRITION DATA PER SERVING:
102 kcal (425 kJ), CHO 15g, protein 5g, fat 2g.

CURRIED BRUSSELS SPROUTS WITH ALMONDS

SERVES FOUR

- 20 Brussels sprouts, with stems trimmed and slit
- 1 teaspoon margarine
- 2 tablespoons blanched, slivered almonds
- 2 teaspoons water
- 1 small onion, finely diced
- 1 teaspoon curry powder

⏱ 10 minutes

METHOD

1. Drop the Brussels sprouts into a saucepan containing 2cm boiling water and boil rapidly for about five minutes, or until cooked, but still firm.
2. Dry the saucepan and return to heat.
3. Melt margarine in saucepan, add almonds and toss until lightly brown. Remove from pan.
4. Add water, onion, and curry powder and stir until onions are lightly cooked.
5. Return sprouts and almonds to saucepan, toss to mix and serve.

NUTRITION DATA PER SERVING:
75 kcal (312 kJ), CHO 3g, protein 5g, fat 5g.

SALADS

All the salad ideas we give here are simple, but show you that with a little inspiration a salad can add something special to a meal. All these recipes will serve four.

Tossed salad

Use your imagination in creating tossed salads. For instance, consider blanched green beans, courgettes, broccoli and cauliflower florets. You can combine alfalfa sprouts, mushrooms, snow peas, sugar-snap peas, carrot and celery with the more traditional ingredients such as various kinds of lettuce, capsicum (bell pepper), cucumber and tomatoes. Avocado adds a certain richness. Toss your choice of ingredients in ¼ cup (60ml) Italian dressing (see recipe, page 168) or an oil-free dressing.

Asparagus and green bean salad

Trim eight spears of fresh asparagus and cut into 7cm lengths. Top, tail and halve 12 green beans. Boil, steam or microwave until just tender, then drop into icy water to cool quickly. (This helps retain their crispness and colour.) Drain. Tear a lettuce into pieces and line a salad bowl. Combine the asparagus, beans and 16 cherry tomatoes and place in the salad bowl. Pour over ¼ cup (60ml) Italian dressing (see recipe, page 168) and sprinkle with 2 tablespoons of toasted sesame seeds.

Ginger carrots

Slice two medium carrots into long strips with a potato peeler. Add a little peeled and finely chopped fresh ginger and pour on ½ cup (125ml) vinegar. Refrigerate for two hours before serving.

Tomato and onion

Slice three firm, ripe tomatoes and a white onion. Pour on ½ cup (125ml) brown vinegar. Add freshly ground black pepper. Refrigerate for at least ½ hour before serving.

Tomato and mint

Mix one ripe, finely chopped tomato with two sliced spring onions and 2 teaspoons chopped, fresh mint. Chill until ready to serve.

Orange and cucumber salad

Peel and slice two oranges, removing all pith. Slice half a cucumber and a small onion. Break the onion into separate rings. Mix orange, cucumber and onion and sprinkle with 1 tablespoon of chopped parsley and, finally, pour over one quantity of creamy orange dressing (see recipe, page 170). Chill well before serving.

Mushroom salad

Slice 10 medium mushrooms into a bowl. Add 1 cup (90g) beanshoots, ½ cup (60g) each celery and red capsicum, cut into matchsticks, and two chopped spring onions. Toss with half a quantity of orange and soy dressing (see recipe, page 169) or herbed tomato dressing (see recipe, page 169) and chill well.

Avocado, spinach and tofu Salad

Wash a bunch of spinach, remove the stalks and tear the leaves into bite-size pieces. Place spinach in a bowl and add a sliced medium avocado, eight pitted and quartered black olives and 250g firm tofu (soybean curd) cut into small cubes. Make a dressing of 2 teaspoons of olive oil, 1 tablespoon lemon juice and a crushed clove of garlic, pour it over the salad and toss lightly. Chill.

Broccoli, beanshoots and snow peas with lemon

Blanch 2 cups (150g) broccoli florets by cooking in boiling water or steaming for three minutes. Plunge quickly under cold water to cool. Steam 12–15 (150g) snow peas for one to two minutes and cool quickly under cold water. Rinse 1 cup (90g) beanshoots and combine with the broccoli and snow peas in a bowl. Pour over a dressing made of 2 tablespoons lemon juice, ½ teaspoon coarsely ground black pepper and 2 teaspoons oil. Serve chilled.

RAITA

SERVES FOUR

- ◆ ¼ cucumber
- ◆ pinch of salt
- ◆ 1 medium tomato
- ◆ 1 small onion
- ◆ 200g low-fat natural yoghurt
- ◆ ¼ teaspoon minced garlic
- ◆ 3–4 drops Tabasco sauce or chilli sauce

⏱ 2 hours

METHOD

1. Peel and chop the cucumber. Sprinkle with salt. Place in sieve over bowl and allow to drain for 30 minutes.
2. Chop tomato and place in the second bowl.
3. Slice onion very finely.
4. Mix tomato, onion and cucumber.
5. Mix yoghurt, garlic and Tabasco or chilli sauce.
6. Pour yoghurt mixture over vegetables, mix well, and refrigerate for one hour.

NUTRITION DATA PER SERVING:
42 kcal (174 kJ), CHO 6g, protein 3g, fat 1g.

SPINACH VALENTINO

SERVES FOUR

- ◆ 1 bunch spinach
- ◆ 4 mushrooms, sliced
- ◆ 2 spring onions, sliced
- ◆ 2 eggs, hard-boiled and sliced
- ◆ 1 quantity orange and soy dressing (see recipe, page 169)

⏱ 5 minutes

METHOD

1. Wash spinach thoroughly, and shake gently to remove excess water. Remove the stalks and tear into bite-size pieces.
2. Combine spinach, mushrooms, spring onions and eggs and toss in dressing.
3. Chill before serving.

NUTRITION DATA PER SERVING:
63 kcal (266 kJ), CHO 2g, protein 5g, fat 4g.

CURRIED PASTA SALAD

SERVES FOUR

- 1½ cups (240g) shell pasta (conchiglie)
- ½ cup (60g) diced celery
- 4 spring onions, chopped
- 2 tablespoons sultanas
- ½ green capsicum (bell pepper), diced
- 2 tablespoons chopped parsley
- ½ cup (80g) corn kernels
- ½ quantity curry dressing (see recipe, page 168)

⏱ 1 hour 15 minutes

METHOD

1. Cook pasta in boiling water for 10–12 minutes until al dente (tender), drain and then run cold water over to cool.
2. Combine pasta, celery, spring onions, sultanas, capsicum, parsley and corn.
3. Toss in curry dressing.
4. Refrigerate for one hour before serving.

NUTRITION DATA PER SERVING:
133 kcal (556 kJ), CHO 26g, protein 5g, fat 1g.

FRUITY PASTA SALAD

SERVES FOUR

- 2½ cups cooked pasta shapes
- ½ cup (85g) sultanas
- 1 stick celery, diced
- 3 spring onions, chopped
- 1 green apple, cored and diced
- 4 dried apricots, chopped
- 4 dried peaches, chopped
- ⅓ cup (50g) pine nuts
- ½ cup (125ml) orange juice
- 1 clove garlic, crushed
- 1 teaspoon minced ginger
- 1 teaspoon lemon juice
- 1 sachet Candarel™ or other sweetener equivalent to 2 teaspoons sugar

⏱ 15 minutes

METHOD

1. Combine pasta, sultanas, celery, spring onions, apple, apricots and peaches in a salad bowl.
2. Toast pine nuts until golden brown in a moderate 180°C (350°F) oven for five to eight minutes. Cool and then add to ingredients in salad bowl.
3. Combine the orange juice, garlic, ginger, lemon juice and sweetener in a screw-top jar, shake well and pour over salad.
4. Toss salad, cover and refrigerate for several hours before serving.

NUTRITION DATA PER SERVING:
327 kcal (1368 kJ), CHO 56g, protein 9g, fat 8g.

BROAD BEAN AND SMOKED SALMON SALAD

SERVES FOUR

- 250g broad beans, frozen or fresh
- 85g smoked salmon, thinly sliced
- 12 cherry tomatoes, halved
- 1 small white onion, thinly sliced
- 2 tablespoons lemon juice
- 2 teaspoons olive oil
- 2 teaspoons capers, drained
- 2 teaspoons chopped fresh parsley

⏱ 20 minutes

METHOD

1. Cook broad beans until they are soft but still retain their shape.
2. Combine broad beans, smoked salmon, cherry tomatoes and onion in a bowl.
3. Blend all the other ingredients in a screw top jar and pour over the salad.
4. Chill and serve.

NUTRITION DATA PER SERVING:
99 kcal (414 kJ), CHO 3g, protein 10g, fat 4g.

FETTUCCINE SALMON SALAD

SERVES FOUR

- 4 cups (1 litre) water
- 250g fresh spinach fettuccine
- 6 spring onions
- ½ stick celery
- ½ capsicum (bell pepper)
- 1 tomato
- ½ courgette
- ½ avocado
- 200g can pink or red salmon
- 1 cup (135g) grated carrot
- 2 tablespoons chopped mint
- juice ½ lemon
- juice 1 orange
- 2 teaspoons olive oil
- 2 teaspoons soy sauce

⏱ 45 minutes

METHOD

1. Heat water until boiling. Add fettuccine and cook until al dente (tender). Drain, rinse and cool.
2. Chop spring onions, celery, capsicum and tomato.
3. Cut courgette into fine strips.
4. Peel avocado and roughly chop.
5. Drain salmon, remove bones and skin.
6. Combine pasta with vegetables and salmon and mix gently.
7. Mix mint, lemon juice, orange juice, olive oil and soy sauce.

NUTRITION DATA PER SERVING:
284 kcal (1189 kJ), CHO 25g, protein 16g, fat 13g.

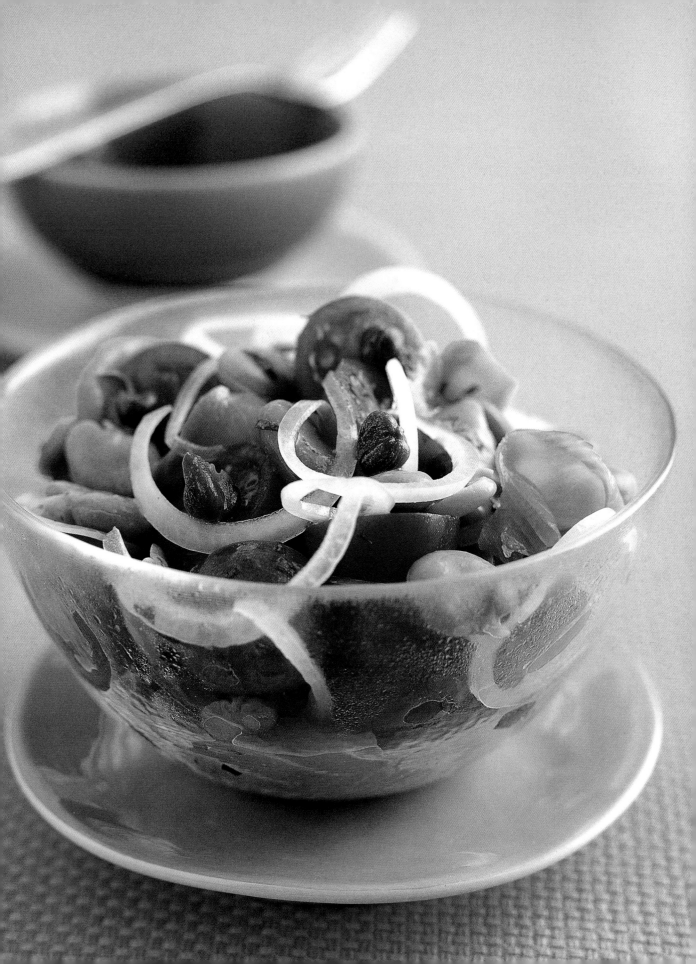

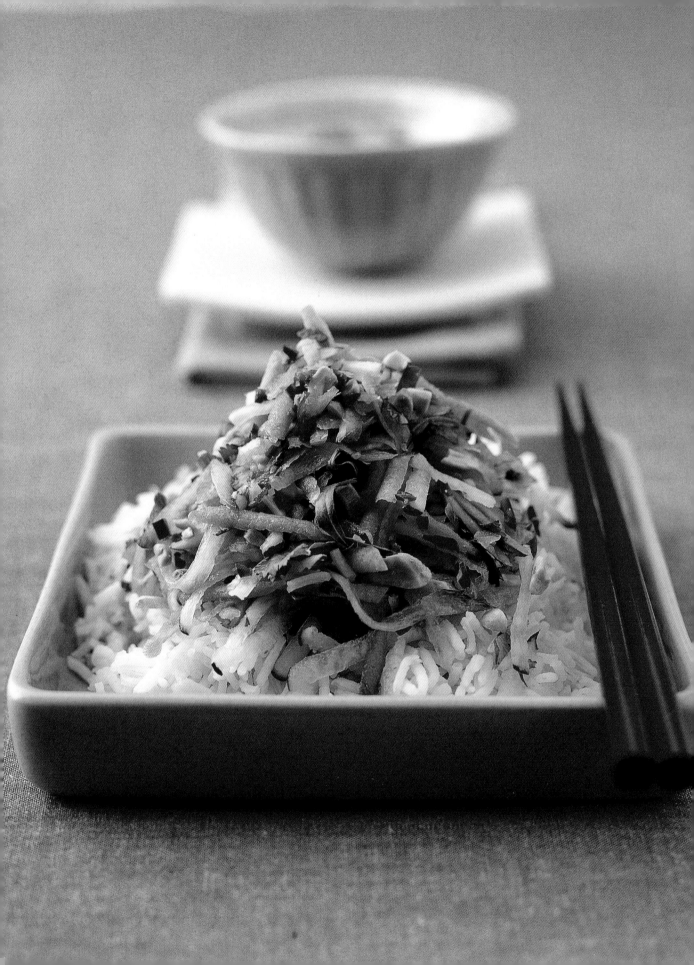

HOT THAI SALAD

SERVES FOUR

- ◆ 2 medium carrots, peeled and grated
- ◆ 1 bunch radish, grated
- ◆ ½ large continental cucumber, grated
- ◆ ⅓ bunch coriander, roughly chopped
- ◆ 2 tablespoons soy sauce
- ◆ 2 tablespoons fish sauce
- ◆ 2 tablespoons mirin
- ◆ 3 tablespoons lemon juice
- ◆ 2 small hot red chillies, seeded and finely chopped

⏱ 10 minutes

METHOD

1. Toss all vegetables together in a large bowl.
2. Place soy sauce, fish sauce, mirin, lemon juice and chillies in a screw top jar and shake well.
3. Pour dressing over salad.
4. Serve on bed of warm rice and top with a sprinkle of chopped nuts or strips of lightly sautéd beef, chicken, pork or seafood.

NUTRITION DATA PER SERVING:
39 kcal (162 kJ), CHO 6g, protein 3g, fat trace.

CRUNCHY RICE SALAD

SERVES FOUR

- ◆ 2 cups (380g) cooked basmati rice
- ◆ ½ green capsicum (bell pepper), chopped
- ◆ ½ red capsicum (bell pepper), chopped
- ◆ 4 spring onions, sliced
- ◆ 4 radishes, finely sliced
- ◆ 1 stick celery, finely sliced
- ◆ ¼ cup (40g) unsalted roasted peanuts
- ◆ ½ cup (80g) canned water chestnuts, drained and sliced
- ◆ ½ cup (60g) green beans, blanched
- ◆ 1 tablespoon soy sauce
- ◆ 1 teaspoon sugar
- ◆ 2 tablespoons chopped parsley
- ◆ ½ cup (45g) bean sprouts
- ◆ pinch of salt (optional)

⏱ 30 minutes

METHOD

1. Combine all ingredients.
2. Chill.
3. Serve garnished with chopped spring onions and radish slices.

NUTRITION DATA PER SERVING:
215 kcal (901 kJ), CHO 35g, protein 7g, fat 5g.

HARLEQUIN PASTA SALAD

SERVES FOUR

- 1 cup (160g) shell pasta (conchiglie)
- 1 cup (160g) cooked and diced skinless chicken fillets
- ½ cup (60g) diced celery
- 1 small green capsicum (bell pepper), chopped
- 1 small red capsicum (bell pepper), chopped
- 4 spring onions, chopped
- 1 tablespoon chopped parsley
- ½ cup (85g) sultanas
- black pepper to taste
- ½ quantity curry dressing (see recipe, page 168)
- 4 lettuce cups, for garnish

⏱ 1 hour 30 minutes

Make this salad the day before you want to serve it, so the flavour can develop.

METHOD

1. Place pasta in a saucepan of boiling water. Cook until tender. Drain.
2. Combine cooked pasta, chicken, celery, capsicum, spring onions, parsley, sultanas and black pepper.
3. Mix in the curry dressing.
4. Refrigerate for one hour.
5. Serve in lettuce cups.

NUTRITION DATA PER SERVING:
227 kcal (950 kJ), CHO 34g, protein 16g, fat 3g.

CURRIED SWEET POTATO AND BANANA SALAD

SERVES FOUR

- 3 medium orange sweet potatoes, peeled
- 2 medium bananas
- 1 tablespoon lemon juice
- 2 spring onions, chopped
- 1 quantity curry dressing (see recipe, page 168)

⏱ 20 minutes

METHOD

1. Cut the sweet potato into 2cm cubes.
2. Place in a large saucepan and barely cover with cold water. Bring to the boil, reduce heat and simmer for about 10–12 minutes, or until potato is cooked through, but still holds it shape. Alternatively, microwave on high for five to six minutes.
3. Meanwhile, slice bananas and toss in lemon juice.
4. Drain the cooked potato and allow to cool.
5. In a salad bowl place the potato, banana, spring onions and dressing and toss gently to combine.

NUTRITION DATA PER SERVING:
125 kcal (524 kJ), CHO 26g, protein 4g, fat 1g.

TANGY POTATO SALAD

SERVES FOUR

- 3 medium potatoes, peeled
- 4 spring onions, chopped
- 3 eggs, hard-boiled and sliced
- ½ cup (125g) low-fat natural yoghurt
- ½ teaspoon black pepper, coarsely ground
- 2 teaspoons curry powder
- 4 lettuce cups

⏱ 30 minutes

This salad is best when made in advance; the flavour develops during refrigeration.

METHOD
1. Cook potatoes until slightly soft, but do not overcook as potato will not hold its shape. Drain.
2. Cut potato into cubes and mix with spring onion. Add eggs.
3. Combine yoghurt, pepper and curry powder. Spoon over the potato mixture and toss gently.
4. Store in airtight container in refrigerator until required.
5. Serve in lettuce cups.

NUTRITION DATA PER SERVING:
131 kcal (550 kJ), CHO 14g, protein 9g, fat 4g.

NEW POTATO SALAD

SERVES FOUR

- 16 small new potatoes
- 2–3 tablespoons fresh mint, chopped
- 2 tablespoons chopped fresh chives, or 2 tablespoons chopped spring onion
- 200g low-fat natural yoghurt
- ½ teaspoon minced or chopped fresh ginger
- ½ teaspoon minced garlic
- ½ teaspoon prepared mild mustard
- 1 teaspoon lemon juice

⏱ 2 hours 45 minutes

METHOD
1. Scrub potatoes if necessary but do not peel.
2. Boil, steam or microwave the potatoes until tender. Drain and cool.
3. Place in serving bowl and add mint and chives or spring onions.
4. In a small mixing bowl combine yoghurt, ginger, garlic, mustard and lemon Juice. Mix well.
5. Pour dressing over potatoes and mix well. Cover and refrigerate until ready to serve.

NUTRITION DATA PER SERVING:
82 kcal (343 kJ), CHO 14g, protein 5g, fat 1g.

COLESLAW

SERVES FOUR

- ¼ medium cabbage, finely shredded
- 1 small onion, grated
- 1 small green capsicum (bell pepper), chopped
- 1 stick celery, chopped
- ⅓ cup (35g) grated carrot
- ground black pepper
- ½ quantity creamy yoghurt dressing (see recipe, page 170)

🕐 10 minutes

VARIATION: Add ⅓ cup chopped pineapple and 2 tablespoons of sultanas. Substitute commercial oil-free coleslaw dressing for creamy yoghurt dressing.

Once you have added the dressing, coleslaw should not be stored. However, you can prepare the vegetables in advance and store them in the refrigerator. Add the dressing just before serving.

METHOD
1. Toss all ingredients in a large bowl and chill until ready to serve.

NUTRITION DATA PER SERVING:
29 kcal (122 kJ), CHO 5g, protein 2g, fat trace.

TABBOULEH

SERVES FOUR

- ½ cup (90g) burghul (cracked wheat)
- 2 large ripe tomatoes, skinned and finely chopped
- 1 small onion, finely chopped
- 1 cup (60g) chopped parsley
- ground black pepper
- 2 teaspoons olive oil
- 2 tablespoons lemon juice
- 1 tablespoon finely chopped mint

🕐 3 hours 15 minutes

METHOD:
1. Place burghul in a deep bowl, cover with boiling water and allow to stand for 2 hours.
2. Drain well by squeezing in a clean muslin cloth or tea towel, and return to bowl.
3. Add the tomatoes, onion, parsley, pepper, oil, lemon juice and mint.
4. Combine well and chill for one hour before serving.

NUTRITION DATA PER SERVING:
112 kcal (470 kJ), CHO 17g, protein 4g, fat 3g.

SAUCES AND DRESSINGS

Sauces and dressings add the final touch to many dishes, but traditionally many are high in fat. We have designed our sauce and dressing recipes to tantalise your taste buds without the fat. Some are based on old-time favourites, but others are new flavour combinations, which we hope will show you that flavoursome dishes do not depend on the use of fats and oils. They can be made so easily and quickly that you will be unable to resist adding them to the repetoire of family favourites!

QUICK AND EASY RELISHES

Banana and yoghurt

Slice 2 firm bananas and sprinkle with 1 tablespoon shredded coconut. Spoon ¼ cup (60g) low-fat yoghurt over bananas and combine. Chill until ready to serve.

Cucumber and yoghurt

Combine a sliced/diced piece of cucumber (about 10cm long) with 2 teaspoons lemon juice and ½ teaspoon mustard seeds. Spoon ¼ cup (60g) low-fat natural yoghurt over the cucumber and stir to combine. Chill until ready to serve.

QUICK AND EASY MARINADES

Try these marinades with lean beef steaks, lamb cutlets, pork schnitzel or as a marinade for meat to place on skewers. They are excellent for barbecues or grills. These quantities are for 500g of meat and will serve four. Stir ingredients, and use to brush meat as it grills.

Red wine zap

Combine ½ cup (125ml) dry red wine, 1 tablespoon tomato purée, 1 tablespoon Worcestershire (or soy, or teriyaki) sauce, 2 tablespoons finely chopped parsley, 1 clove crushed garlic, ground black pepper to taste and ¼ teaspoon finely chopped oregano or basil (optional). To 'rev it up', add ¼ cup (60ml) sweet chilli sauce, ¼ cup (60ml) Worcestershire sauce, or 1–2 cloves crushed garlic.

Singapore sizzler

Combine 1 tablespoon Worcestershire sauce, 1 tablespoon soy or teriyaki sauce, 2 tablespoons lemon juice, ¼ teaspoon mustard powder, ¼ teaspoon ground coriander and ¼ teaspoon finely chopped fresh ginger.

Spicy lamb

Particularly good for lamb is a combination of ½ cup (125ml) tomato purée, 2 teaspoons Worcestershire sauce, 2 teaspoons chopped fresh or ½ teaspoon dried rosemary, dash of Tabasco sauce and four chopped spring onions.

WHITE SAUCE

MAKES 2 CUPS

- ◆ 2 cups (500ml) skimmed milk
- ◆ 1 onion, cut in half
- ◆ 1 small carrot, roughly chopped
- ◆ 1 stalk celery, roughly chopped
- ◆ 6 peppercorns
- ◆ 2 tablespoons cornflour (cornstarch)

⏱ 20 minutes

METHOD

1. Pour milk into saucepan. Add chopped vegetables and peppercorns.
2. Bring mixture to boil. Immediately reduce heat and simmer for 15 minutes.
3. Strain milk into a bowl. Discard vegetables and peppercorns.
4. In a separate bowl, mix cornflour with 2 or 3 tablespoons of the warm milk. Stir to make a smooth paste.
5. Gradually add remaining milk to the paste, stirring all the time.
6. Return sauce to the saucepan. Bring to boil, stirring constantly. Reduce heat and simmer gently for two minutes, stirring until sauce thickens.
7. Use as required in recipes.

NUTRITION DATA PER TOTAL QUANTITY:
247 kcal (1036 kJ), CHO 40g, protein 20g, fat 1g.

CHERRY SAUCE

MAKES 2 CUPS

- ◆ 2 cups (300g) fresh ripe cherries, pitted
- ◆ ½ cup chicken stock (see recipe, page 68) or ½ cup (125ml) water and 1 stock cube
- ◆ 1 teaspoon Worcestershire sauce
- ◆ 1 tablespoon brandy

⏱ 15 minutes

METHOD

1. Place 1 cup of cherries into a saucepan or in a microwave bowl with stock and Worcestershire sauce.
2. Boil for eight minutes until cherries are soft, or microwave on high for four minutes. Purée and return to saucepan or bowl.
3. Add remaining cup of cherries and brandy. Simmer for two minutes or microwave on high for two minutes, and serve.

NUTRITION DATA PER TOTAL QUANTITY:
192 kcal (804 kJ), CHO 48g, protein 2g, fat 0g.

CHEESE SAUCE

MAKES 2 CUPS

- ◆ 250g cottage or ricotta cheese
- ◆ ½ cup (60g) grated reduced-fat cheddar cheese
- ◆ ½ cup (125ml) skimmed milk
- ◆ 1 tablespoon cornflour (cornstarch)
- ◆ 1 tablespoon skimmed milk, extra

⏱ 10 minutes

VARIATION: If you'd like a little more 'bite', add ½ teaspoon prepared English mustard and a pinch of cayenne pepper.

METHOD

1. Using a food processor or electric blender, blend ricotta or cottage cheese and skimmed milk until smooth. Add the grated cheese.
2. In saucepan, gently warm the cheese mixture, stirring constantly, until the grated cheese melts.
3. In a cup, blend the cornflour with the extra tablespoon of milk to make a smooth paste. Add to saucepan and stir into sauce.
4. Stirring constantly, bring sauce to the boil. Immediately reduce heat and simmer gently for two minutes, stirring constantly.

NUTRITION DATA PER TOTAL QUANTITY:
498 kcal (2084 kJ), CHO 21g, protein 66g, fat 18g.

SATAY (PEANUT) SAUCE

MAKES 2 CUPS

- ◆ 1 tablespoon water
- ◆ 1 small onion, grated
- ◆ 1 clove garlic, crushed
- ◆ ½–1 teaspoon ground chilli
- ◆ ¾ cup (230g) crunchy peanut butter (preferably low-salt)
- ◆ 1 tablespoon soy sauce
- ◆ 1 tablespoon lemon juice
- ◆ 1¼ cups (300ml) water

⏱ 20 minutes

METHOD

1. In a frying pan, bring water to the boil. Add onion and garlic and cook gently until soft.
2. Add chilli, stir in and cook for one minute over medium heat.
3. Add peanut butter and stir well. Add soy sauce, lemon juice and water and mix well. Bring mixture to boil, stirring constantly. Reduce heat and simmer gently for one minute.

NUTRITION DATA PER TOTAL QUANTITY:
370 kcal (1548 kJ), CHO 9g, protein 14g, fat 32g.

FRESH VEGETABLE SAUCE

MAKES 4 CUPS

- 1 apple, peeled and grated
- 1 medium courgette, grated
- ¼ medium green capsicum (bell pepper), finely chopped
- 1 small onion, finely chopped
- 2 medium tomatoes, finely chopped
- 3 medium mushrooms, finely chopped
- 1 medium carrot, grated
- 1 clove garlic, crushed
- 1 tablespoon finely chopped parsley
- ½ teaspoon finely chopped fresh sage, or ¼ teaspoon dried sage
- ½ teaspoon finely chopped fresh marjoram or ¼ teaspoon dried marjoram
- ground black pepper
- 2 tablespoons tomato paste
- ½ cup (125ml) water

⏲ 30 minutes

METHOD

1. Place all ingredients in saucepan, bring to the boil and simmer for 20 minutes. Alternatively, place the ingredients in a microwave-proof bowl, and microwave on high for 10 minutes.

NUTRITION DATA PER TOTAL QUANTITY:
221 kcal (927 kJ), CHO 40g, protein 14g, fat 1g.

TOMATO AND BASIL SAUCE

SERVES FOUR

- 2 teaspoon olive oil
- 1 medium onion, finely chopped
- 1 clove garlic, crushed
- 500g ripe tomatoes, peeled, seeded and chopped
- 1 tablespoon chopped fresh basil
- ½ teaspoon chopped fresh oregano
- ground black pepper

⏲ 20 minutes

METHOD

1. Heat oil in saucepan, add onion and sauté until translucent.
2. Add garlic and cook for a further two minutes.
3. Add tomatoes, herbs and pepper and boil for eight to ten minutes.
4. Alternatively, if you prefer to use the microwave, sauté onion in the microwave until soft (approximately 30 seconds). Add garlic and cook on high for a further minute. Add the tomatoes, herbs and pepper, and cook on high for four to six minutes.

NUTRITION DATA PER TOTAL QUANTITY:
190 kcal (793 kJ), CHO 19g, protein 6g, fat 10g.

BLACK BEAN SAUCE

MAKES ½ CUP

- 3 tablespoons dried black beans, soaked overnight, or canned
- 1 clove garlic, crushed
- ½ teaspoon finely chopped or minced fresh ginger
- 1 tablespoon brandy or dry sherry
- ¼ cup (60ml) water
- 2 teaspoons soy sauce

⏱ 7 minutes

This sauce is delicious with finely sliced sautéed steak, chicken fillets or fish.

METHOD

1. Wash beans thoroughly, drain and mash with garlic, ginger and brandy or sherry.
2. Place in a saucepan with water and soy sauce.
3. Bring to the boil, reduce heat and simmer for two minutes.

NUTRITION DATA PER TOTAL QUANTITY:
183 kcal (767 kJ), CHO 16g, protein 15g, fat 8g.

RATATOUILLE SAUCE

SERVES FOUR

- 1 small green capsicum (bell pepper), diced
- 1 small aubergine, peeled and diced
- 2 small courgettes, diced
- 2 medium tomatoes, diced, or 16 cherry tomatoes
- 6 medium mushrooms, diced
- 1 large onion, peeled and diced
- 1 clove garlic, crushed
- ½ teaspoon dried oregano
- black pepper to taste
- 3 tablespoons water

⏱ 45 minutes

Ratatouille can be served hot or chilled as a salad. It is also ideal used to surround chicken, veal or fish fillets during cooking.

METHOD

1. Combine all ingredients and cook over low heat for 30 minutes, or microwave on medium for 15 minutes.

NUTRITION DATA PER TOTAL QUANTITY:
44 kcal (184 kJ), CHO 7g, protein 4g, fat 1g.

CUCUMBER AND YOGHURT SAUCE

MAKES 1 CUP

- ½ cucumber, peeled
- 200g low-fat natural yoghurt
- 1 teaspoon finely chopped or minced fresh ginger
- ½ teaspoon minced garlic
- 1 tablespoon lemon juice
- ¼ teaspoon freshly ground black pepper
- ¼ teaspoon mild paprika
- 1 tablespoon chopped parsley
- 4 cardamom pods, crushed

⏱ 15 minutes

Use this sauce straightaway because it will not keep.

METHOD
1. Grate cucumber, drain well and discard liquid.
2. Combine all the ingredients in a bowl and chill well before serving.

NUTRITION DATA PER TOTAL QUANTITY:
123 kcal (514 kJ), CHO 16g, protein 11g, fat 2g.

STRAWBERRY AND PEPPERCORN SAUCE

MAKES 2 CUPS

- ½ cup (125ml) dry white wine
- ½ punnet strawberries, washed, hulled and puréed
- 1 teaspoon lemon juice
- 1 teaspoon brandy
- 2 teaspoons green or pink peppercorns
- ½ cup (125ml) canned evaporated skimmed milk, chilled

⏱ 15 minutes

Unusual, but wonderful with grilled or sautéed chicken fillets, fish, lobster or crab.

METHOD
1. Bring wine to the boil and reduce to half by simmering.
2. Add strawberry purée, lemon juice, brandy and peppercorns.
3. Bring back to the boil, simmer for one minute and set aside to cool.
4. Whip milk until it is thick. Gradually add the strawberry mixture, whipping constantly.
5. Gently reheat the mixture, but do not allow it to boil. Serve immediately.

NUTRITION DATA PER TOTAL QUANTITY:
48 kcal (200 kJ), CHO 7g, protein 5g, fat trace.

SWEET AND SOUR SAUCE

SERVES FOUR

- 1 large onion
- 8 spring onions
- 2 medium carrots
- 1 small red capsicum
  (bell pepper), de-seeded
- 125g mushrooms
- 2 sticks celery
- 1 medium cucumber
- 2 teaspoon oil
- 1 clove garlic, crushed
- 1 teaspoon grated or minced
  fresh ginger
- 2 tablespoons tomato purée
- ¼ cup (60ml) white vinegar
- 1 cup (250ml) water
- 1 stock cube
- 1½ tablespoons cornflour
  (cornstarch)
- 3 tablespoons soy sauce
- 1 tablespoon dry sherry
- 400g can unsweetened
  pineapple pieces and juice

⏱ 30 minutes

This is a wonderfully versatile sauce that is just as good served with boiled brown rice or noodles, as it is served with grilled fish, pork or vegetables.

METHOD

1. Slice onion, spring onions, capsicum, mushrooms and celery thinly (about matchstick size).
2. Cut cucumber into quarters, lengthwise, remove seeds and cut into small pieces of about 1½ cm.
3. Heat oil in a large wok or frying pan over high heat. Add garlic and ginger. Stir-fry for 30 seconds, and then add all the other vegetables. Keep heat high and stir-fry for two to three minutes until the vegetables are cooked, but still crisp and bright coloured.
4. In a bowl, blend tomato purée, vinegar, water, stock cube, cornflour, soy sauce and sherry.
5. Drain pineapple pieces, and add the juice to the tomato paste mixture. Keep pineapple aside. Add sauce mixture to the vegetables, and stir until sauce boils and thickens.
6. Add pineapple to the vegetables, and cook for another three to five minutes until the pineapple is heated through.
7. Serve hot or cold as an accompaniment with grilled fish, or pork and vegetables en brochette (see recipe, page 141). As a light meal, serve the sauce with boiled brown rice or noodles.

NUTRITION DATA PER TOTAL QUANTITY:
517 kcal (2163 kJ), CHO 87g, protein 17g, fat 11g.

GREEN CHAMPAGNE SAUCE

MAKES 1 CUP

- ◆ 3 kiwifruit, peeled and puréed
- ◆ ½ cup (85g) halved sultana grapes
- ◆ ½ cup (125ml) champagne

⏱ 10 minutes

Simple, sophisticated and superb, especially with fish.

METHOD
1. Place kiwifruit in saucepan. Add grapes and champagne.
2. Heat gently, but do not boil. Serve immediately.

NUTRITION DATA PER TOTAL QUANTITY:
289 kcal (1210 kJ), CHO 46g, protein 5g, fat 1g.

ITALIAN DRESSING

MAKES ½ CUP

- ◆ ⅓ cup (80ml) vinegar
- ◆ 1 tablespoon lemon juice
- ◆ 1 tablespoon chopped parsley
- ◆ 2 teaspoons chopped chives
- ◆ 1 clove garlic, crushed
- ◆ ½ teaspoon dry mustard
- ◆ ground black pepper

⏱ 5 minutes

METHOD
1. Combine ingredients in a screw top jar, shake well and refrigerate.

NUTRITION DATA PER TOTAL QUANTITY:
negligible.

CURRY DRESSING

MAKES ½ CUP

- ◆ ½ cup (125ml) low-fat natural yoghurt
- ◆ 2 teaspoons hot curry powder or paste (see recipes, page 171)
- ◆ 2 tablespoons chopped parsley
- ◆ ¼ teaspoon minced garlic (optional)

⏱ 5 minutes

METHOD
1. Mix all ingredients and adjust flavourings to taste.
2. Chill and use same day.

NUTRITION DATA PER TOTAL QUANTITY:
80 kcal (337 kJ), CHO 9g, protein 8g, fat 2g.

ORANGE AND SOY DRESSING

MAKES ¼ CUP

- ¼ cup (60ml) unsweetened orange juice
- 2 teaspoons soy sauce
- 1 clove garlic, crushed
- 1 teaspoon oil (optional)

⏱ 5 minutes

METHOD
1. Combine all ingredients in a screw top jar.
2. Chill and shake well before use.

NUTRITION DATA PER TOTAL QUANTITY:
64 kcal (269 kJ), CHO 4g, protein trace, fat 5g.

HERBED TOMATO DRESSING

MAKES 1 CUP

- ½ cup (125ml) unsweetened tomato juice
- 4 tablespoons tomato purée
- 2 tablespoons low-fat natural yoghurt
- 4 drops Tabasco sauce
- 1 clove garlic, crushed
- 1 tablespoon chopped parsley
- ½ teaspoon chopped fresh mixed herbs, e.g. marjoram, basil or thyme, or ½ teaspoon mixed dried herbs.

⏱ 8 minutes

METHOD
1. Combine tomato juice with tomato purée and add to yoghurt.
2. Add other ingredients and mix well.
3. Chill and use same day.

NUTRITION DATA PER TOTAL QUANTITY:
98 kcal (411 kJ), CHO 16g, protein 8g, fat trace.

CREAMY YOGHURT DRESSING

MAKES ½ CUP

- ⅓ cup (80ml) low-fat natural yoghurt
- 2 tablespoons lemon juice or raspberry vinegar
- ½ teaspoon dry mustard
- ground black pepper

⏱ 5 minutes

METHOD

1. Mix all ingredients until smooth. Cover and refrigerate.

NUTRITION DATA PER TOTAL QUANTITY:
45 kcal (189 kJ), CHO 6g, protein 4g, fat 1g.

CREAMY ORANGE DRESSING

MAKES ¾ CUP

- ¼ cup (60ml) unsweetened orange juice
- 2 teaspoons grated orange rind
- 1 tablespoon finely chopped parsley
- 2 teaspoons finely chopped chives
- ½ cup (125g) low-fat natural yoghurt

⏱ 5 minutes

VARIATION: For creamy lemon dressing, prepare as above but omit orange juice and rind, replacing them with 2 tablespoons lemon juice.

METHOD

1. Combine all ingredients and chill.

NUTRITION DATA PER TOTAL QUANTITY:
101 kcal (421 kJ), CHO 14g, protein 8g, fat 2g.

CURRY PASTE

MAKES ¼ CUP

- 1 tablespoon freshly minced or grated ginger
- 2 tablespoons ground coriander
- 1 tablespoon ground cinnamon
- 2 teaspoons chilli powder
- 1 tablespoon powdered turmeric
- 1 teaspoon minced garlic
- 1 tablespoon lemon juice
- 2 tablespoons vinegar
- 2 tablespoons oil
- 1 tablespoon seeded mustard

⏱ 6 minutes

You can vary the quantities and ingredients of this curry paste according to taste.

METHOD

1. Combine ingredients in saucepan and mix to make a smooth paste.
2. Stirring constantly, cook over low heat for three to four minutes until slightly thickened.
3. Spoon mixture into a warmed glass jar, seal and store in refrigerator.

NUTRITION DATA PER TOTAL QUANTITY:
negligible.

CURRY POWDER

MAKES ¼ CUP

- ½ teaspoon cayenne pepper
- 2 tablespoons ground coriander
- 1 tablespoon ground cumin
- 1 tablespoon coarsely ground black pepper
- 2 tablespoons ground ginger
- 1 tablespoon ground cinnamon
- ½ teaspoon ground cloves
- ¼ teaspoon ground nutmeg
- 2 teaspoons chilli powder
- 2 tablespoons powdered turmeric

⏱ 15 minutes

You can vary the ingredients and quantities according to taste. Curry powder can be stored for a long time, but gradually loses its flavour.

METHOD

1. Mix ingredients well.
2. Refrigerate in airtight container.

NUTRITION DATA PER TOTAL QUANTITY:
negligible.

TOMATO RELISH

MAKES 3.5 LITRES

- 3 large onions
- 2½kg chopped, ripe tomatoes
- 5 granny smith apples, cored and chopped (skins left on)
- 3 cups (750ml) vinegar
- 500g sultanas
- 3 cloves of garlic, crushed
- 1 cup (250ml) fresh orange juice
- 1 teaspoon mixed spice
- 4 whole cloves
- 1 teaspoon chilli powder

⏱ 1 hour 30 minutes

METHOD

1. Place all the ingredients in a large saucepan and bring to the boil. Turn the heat to low and simmer for one hour, stirring frequently. Remove from heat.
2. Pour hot water into clean jars to warm them. Pour water away.
3. Fill jars with hot chutney. Allow them to cool, then seal the jars and store.

NUTRITION DATA PER TOTAL QUANTITY:
2107 kcal (8820 kJ), CHO 503g, protein 42g, fat 1g.

FRESH MANGO PICKLE

MAKES ¼–1 CUP

- 1 ripe medium-large mango
- 2 teaspoons lemon juice
- ½ teaspoon finely chopped or minced fresh ginger
- 1 tablespoon sultanas

⏱ 15 minutes

METHOD

1. Peel mango. Slice flesh from stone and cut into small pieces. Place in a mixing bowl.
2. Add lemon juice, ginger, and sultanas.
3. Spoon into glass or plastic container, cover and refrigerate.

NUTRITION DATA PER TOTAL QUANTITY:
102 kcal (425 kJ), CHO 24g, protein 2g, fat trace.

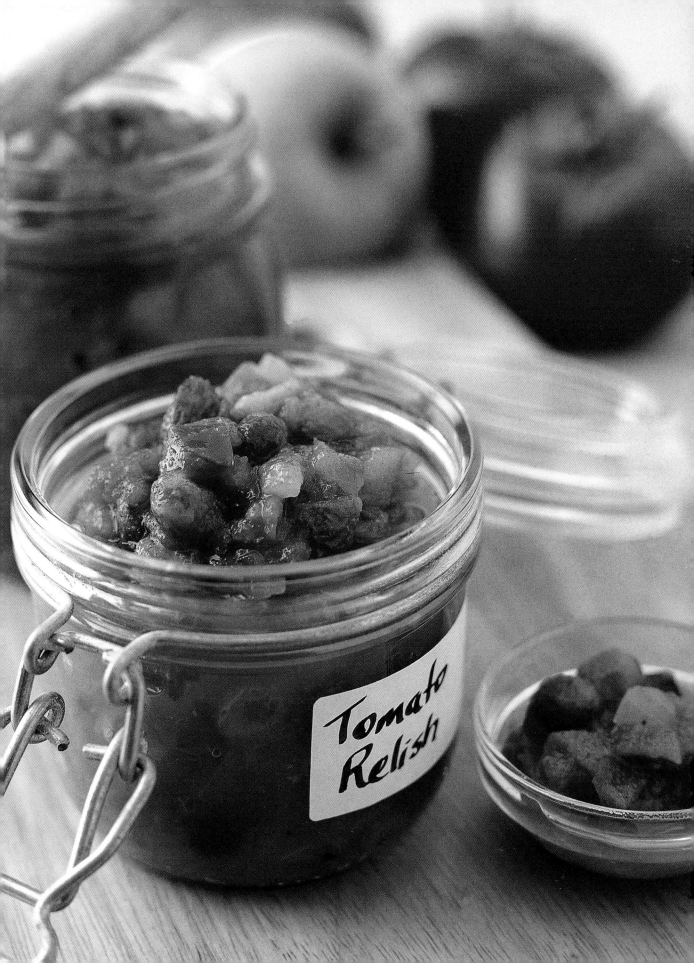

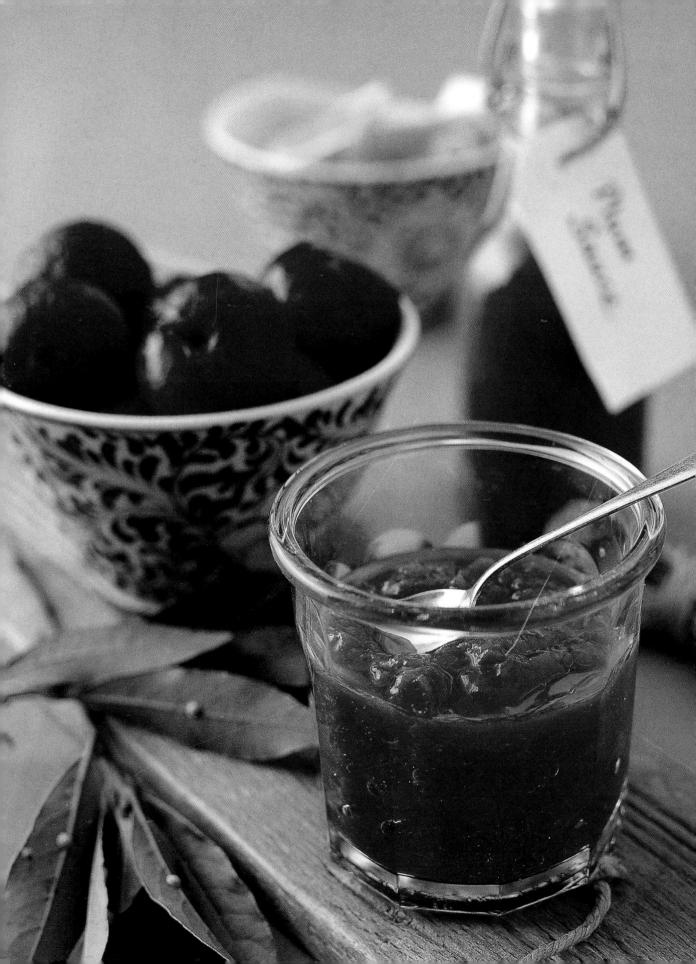

PLUM SAUCE

MAKES 1 LITRE

- 2 onions, chopped
- 1 cup (250ml) water
- 1 kg (2lb) fresh plums, stoned
- 1 cup (250ml) fresh orange juice
- 2 teaspoons grated or minced fresh ginger
- ½ teaspoon whole cloves
- ¼ teaspoon peppercorns
- pinch of thyme
- pinch of oregano
- 1 bay leaf

⏱ 1 hour 30 minutes

METHOD

1. Lightly sauté onions in 2–3 tablespoons of the water, for two minutes.
2. Add the rest of the ingredients and cook over low heat, stirring regularly.
3. Simmer, with the lid off, for at least one hour until the mixture thickens.
4. Pour into clean warmed jars, allow to cool and then seal.

NUTRITION DATA PER TOTAL QUANTITY:
545 kcal (2238 kJ), CHO 124g, protein 12g, fat 1g.

BLUEBERRY SAUCE

SERVES FOUR

- 1 cup (160g) blueberries, fresh or frozen
- ½ cup (125ml) orange juice
- ½ teaspoon cinnamon
- 1 tablespoon brown sugar
- 2 teaspoons cornflour (cornstarch)
- 1 tablespoon water

⏱ 15 minutes

METHOD

1. Place berries, juice, cinnamon, and sugar into a saucepan. Bring orange juice to the boil, then remove from heat.
2. Combine cornflour and water, making sure there are no lumps.
3. Stir into the berries, then reheat until the mixture thickens.
4. Spoon hot sauce over pancakes.

NUTRITION DATA PER SERVING:
52 kcal (217 kJ), CHO 13g, protein 0.4 g, fat trace.

CUSTARD SAUCE

SERVES FOUR

- 3 level tablespoons custard powder
- 2 cups (500 ml) skimmed milk
- 1 teaspoon vanilla
- 2 teaspoons sugar, Candarel™ or other artificial sweetener

⏱ 15 minutes

VARIATION: Add 1 teaspoon of finely grated orange rind to milk before heating.

You can serve this sauce hot or cold.

METHOD

1. Blend custard powder and a small quantity of the milk to make a smooth paste.
2. Place remaining milk in saucepan and bring to boil.
3. Gradually stir in custard paste. Continue stirring until mixture thickens.
4. Simmer for one minute, stirring constantly.
5. Add vanilla and sugar, Candarel™ or other artificial sweetener.

NUTRITION DATA PER SERVING:
71 kcal (298 kJ), CHO 13g, protein 5g, fat trace.

BRANDY SAUCE

SERVES FOUR

- 1 quantity of custard sauce (see recipe above)
- 1 egg, separated
- 2 tablespoons brandy

⏱ 20 minutes

METHOD

1. Beat egg yolk and add to custard sauce.
2. Whip egg white until peaks form.
3. Fold egg white through custard and add brandy.
4. Serve immediately.

NUTRITION DATA PER SERVING:
110 kcal (462 kJ), CHO 13g, protein 6g, fat 1g.

DESSERTS

In this section we show you that desserts do not need to be loaded with cream and sugar to be enticing. We have designed the dessert recipes in this section to be nutritious components of a meal. For example, fruits and dairy foods, which are mainly low glycaemic index foods, add vitamins and minerals as well as the all-important carbohydrates. With these recipes, as in other sections of the book, we hope to stimulate your imagination. Once you have tried some of these easy and tasty dishes, you will want to branch out and use them as the basis for your own recipe ideas. You can, for example, use different fruits and spices. All are suitable for the whole family and for friends.

Pastries are traditionally high in fat but here we show you how to make a low-fat fruit strudel (see recipe, page 176) using filo pastry. Filo is a fine pastry, originating in Greece, which is almost fat free and adapts well to a variety of uses. Rather than brushing the layers with melted butter as is usual, we use semi-skimmed milk. You can also use a spray oil to separate the layers and maintain crispness without using large amounts of fat or oil. Filo pastry can be readily purchased in the supermarket, either fresh or frozen, although the fresh version, if available, is easier to use. If you have a microwave, use it to help make dessert preparation quick and easy. It can also save on dirty dishes. For example fruit cooks very well in the microwave, and making custard sauce is very much quicker and easier than using a saucepan.

A hint for fruit juice: to get more juice from citrus fruit, first microwave the whole fruit on high for one to two minutes. Stand for 30 seconds, then squeeze out the juice.

APPLE STRUDEL

SERVES FOUR

- 6 sheets filo pastry
- 2 tablespoons skimmed milk, or a little cooking spray
- 4 apples, peeled and sliced very finely
- 4 tablespoons sultanas
- 2 tablespoons chopped pecans or walnuts
- 1 teaspoon cinnamon
- ¼ teaspoon ground cloves
- 1 tablespoon brown sugar

⏱ 45 minutes

All the pleasure of the traditional strudel, but with a fraction of the fat.

METHOD

1. Spread out two sheets of pastry on a kitchen bench. Brush lightly with milk, or spray lightly with cooking spray.
2. Place another two layers of pastry on top. Again brush with milk.
3. Repeat for remaining two sheets of pastry.
4. Sprinkle remaining ingredients over the pastry.
5. Spray a baking tray with non-stick baking spray. Carefully roll up the pastry. Place on the baking tray, loose edge down.
6. Brush the strudel well with milk. Bake in a preheated 200°C (400°F) oven for 25–30 minutes.
7. Serve warm, cut into thick slices.

NUTRITION DATA PER SERVING:
191 kcal (800 kJ), CHO 36g, protein 5g, fat 5g.

Variations

BANANA STRUDEL

For this delectable filling combine four ripe bananas (sliced), 4 tablespoons sultanas, 1 teaspoon cinnamon, 4 tablespoons shredded coconut, 2 tablespoons unsweetened orange juice, 2 tablespoons chopped pecans or walnuts, 4 tablespoons dark rum and 1 teaspoon brown sugar.

NUTRITION DATA PER SERVING:
263 kcal (1102 kJ), CHO 43 g, protein 7g, fat 9g.

APRICOT STRUDEL

For the filling combine 500g apricots (stoned and sliced) or 1 can (425g) of unsweetened apricot pieces, 4 tablespoons sultanas, 2 tablespoons slivered almonds, 1 teaspoon cinnamon and 1 tablespoon brown sugar.

NUTRITION DATA PER SERVING:
138 kcal (580 kJ), CHO 22 g, protein 5g, fat 5g.

FRUIT CRUMBLE

SERVES FOUR

- 3 large cooking apples, peeled cored and sliced
- 2 tablespoons water
- ½ teaspoon ground cinnamon or 3 cloves
- ½ cup (50g) rolled oats
- 2 tablespoons desiccated coconut
- 2 tablespoons mixed dried fruit
- 2 teaspoons chopped nuts
- ¼ cup (25g) wheatflakes
- ¼ (15g) cup All-bran

OR

- 1⅓ cups (130g) Meg's muesli (see recipe, page 56)

⏱ 1 hour

You can replace the apples in this recipe with peaches, apricots or plums or with two apples and half a cup of cooked rhubarb. If you have a favourite combination, you can use it in this recipe, too.

METHOD

1. Place apple into a saucepan, add water and cinnamon or cloves.
2. Simmer gently for approximately 10 minutes until apple is tender, or microwave, covered, on high for six minutes.
3. Lightly grease a small casserole and spoon in apple, removing cloves if used.
4. Mix rolled oats, desiccated coconut, dried fruit, nuts, wheatflakes and All-bran, if using. Sprinkle this topping mixture or Meg's muesli thickly over apple.
5. Bake in a preheated 180°C (350°F) oven for 30 minutes or until topping becomes golden. Serve hot or cold.

NUTRITION DATA PER SERVING:
245 kcal (1025 kJ), CHO 38g, protein 7g, fat 7g.

HOT JAMAICAN PINEAPPLE

SERVES FOUR

- ½ medium pineapple, cut lengthwise with top intact
- 3 bananas, peeled and chopped
- 4 teaspoons dark rum
- 2 teaspoons brown sugar
- ¼ cup (20g) desiccated coconut

⏱ 1 hour

METHOD

1. Cut pineapple out of skin, being careful not to pierce skin. Scoop out any remaining pulp and juice and retain.
2. Chop pineapple into chunks, discarding core. Add to pulp and juice a in bowl. Add bananas, rum and brown sugar.
3. Place in baking dish, sprinkle with coconut and bake in a preheated 180°C (350°F) oven for 30–45 minutes until fruit is heated through and coconut is toasted.
4. Spoon into reserved pineapple skin to serve.

NUTRITION DATA PER SERVING:
130 kcal (542 kJ), CHO 25g, protein 2g, fat 2g.

SWEET POTATO AND PECAN PIE

SERVES EIGHT

- ◆ 15 shredded wheatmeal biscuits, crushed
- ◆ 3 tablespoons margarine, melted
- ◆ 2 cups (470g) mashed cooked sweet potato
- ◆ 4 tablespoons lemon juice
- ◆ 1 teaspoon cinnamon
- ◆ ¼ teaspoon mixed spice
- ◆ ¼ teaspoon ground ginger
- ◆ 3 tablespoons brown sugar
- ◆ pinch salt
- ◆ 1 cup (250ml) semi-skimmed milk
- ◆ 125g pecan kernels
- ◆ 2 eggs, separated

⏱ 1 hour 30 minutes

METHOD

1. Line a pie or flan dish with aluminium foil.
2. Mix crushed biscuits with margarine and spoon into dish. Spread over base and up the sides, pressing with the back of a spoon.
3. Bake in a preheated 180°C (350°F) oven for 10–15 minutes, then remove and cool.
4. Spoon sweet potato into a mixing bowl. Add lemon juice, cinnamon, mixed spice, ginger, sugar, and salt and stir well to combine.
5. Stir in milk, pecan kernels and egg yolks.
6. Beat egg whites until soft peaks form, then fold into sweet potato mixture.
7. Spoon into crumb crust and bake for 45–60 minutes, or until set and lightly browned. Serve warm or cold.

NUTRITION DATA PER PORTION:
344 kcal (1439 kJ), CHO 31g, protein 7g, fat 22g.

MIXED BERRY SALAD WITH LEMON CREAM

SERVES FOUR

- ◆ 1 punnet or 250g strawberries
- ◆ 1 punnet or 250g blackberries
- ◆ 1 punnet or 250g blueberries
- ◆ ¼ cup (60ml) unsweetened apple juice
- ◆ 250g ricotta cheese
- ◆ 100g low-fat natural yoghurt
- ◆ rind of 1 lemon, grated
- ◆ 2 teaspoons brown sugar

⏱ 30 minutes

VARIATION: Replace blackberries with loganberries.

When berries are in season celebrate with this salad, dressed with smooth lemon cream.

METHOD

1. Wash and hull berries and slice strawberries, if large.
2. Place in bowl and pour over the apple juice.
3. Chill in refrigerator.
4. Mix ricotta, yoghurt, lemon rind and sugar. Chill.
5. Spoon lemon cream over fruit and serve.

NUTRITION DATA PER SERVING:
100 kcal (419 kJ), CHO 20g, protein 4g, fat 1g.

PUMPKIN PIE

SERVES SIX

- ◆ 2 tablespoons margarine
- ◆ 1 cup (140g) wholemeal flour
- ◆ 1 egg yolk
- ◆ juice of ½ lemon plus cold water to make ⅓ cup
- ◆ 2 cups (350g) firm pumpkin purée
- ◆ ¼ cup (65g) ricotta cheese
- ◆ ¼ cup (60ml) low-fat natural yoghurt
- ◆ ½ cup (125ml) skimmed or semi-skimmed milk
- ◆ 2 eggs, separated
- ◆ ¼ teaspoon nutmeg
- ◆ ¼ teaspoon mixed spice
- ◆ ½ teaspoon cinnamon
- ◆ juice and grated rind of 1 lemon
- ◆ Candarel™ or other artificial sweetener to taste
- ◆ ground cinnamon, for garnish

🕐 2 hours

VARIATION: Fold ¼ cup (30g) chopped pecans into filling.

This is simply delicious.

METHOD
1. Rub margarine into flour until mixture resembles fine breadcrumbs.
2. Mix egg yolk with juice and water.
3. Mix liquid into flour with a knife, to make a soft dough.
4. Turn out onto a floured board. Knead lightly and leave for 15 minutes.
5. Roll out pastry, then use it to cover base and sides of a pie dish. Add a second strip around the top edge and pinch as a decorative edge. Prick pastry and bake in a preheated 180°C (350°F) oven for approximately one hour until lightly browned. Remove and cool.
6. Combine pumpkin, ricotta, yoghurt, milk and egg yolks in a bowl. Beat well.
7. Add spices, lemon juice and rind, and sweetener. Check the taste and adjust if necessary.
8. Beat egg whites until soft peaks form and fold into pumpkin mixture.
9. Pour into pastry shell and bake in the oven until set (about one hour).
10. Sprinkle with a little cinnamon to serve.

NUTRITION DATA PER SERVING:
203 kcal (851 kJ), CHO 20g, protein 9g, fat 10g.

FRUITY BAKED RICE PUDDING

SERVES FOUR

- ◆ 3½ cups (875ml) skimmed milk
- ◆ 5 tablespoons basmati rice
- ◆ 1 tablespoon sugar
- ◆ 4 tablespoons sultanas or raisins
- ◆ 4 tablespoons dried peaches
  or apricots
- ◆ ground nutmeg or cinnamon,
  for garnish

⏱ 2 hours

METHOD

1. Combine milk, rice and sugar.
2. Place mixture in baking dish.
3. Cover and bake in a preheated 180°C (350°F) oven for
   45 minutes.
4. Remove from oven, add dried fruit and stir.
5. Leave uncovered and return to oven. Cook for another
   45–60 minutes until rice is cooked. A skin will form on
   top of rice.
6. Serve hot or cold, garnished with ground nutmeg or
   cinnamon.

NUTRITION DATA PER SERVING:
284 kcal (1191 kJ), CHO 60g, protein 11g, fat trace.

OLD-FASHIONED DUMPLINGS

SERVES FOUR

- ◆ ¾ cup (190ml) skimmed or
  semi-skimmed milk
- ◆ ¼ teaspoon ground nutmeg
- ◆ ½ cup (80g) semolina
- ◆ 1 egg
- ◆ 1 teaspoon vanilla essence
- ◆ 1 tablespoon mixed peel
- ◆ 1 tablespoon currants
- ◆ 1 tablespoon sultanas
- ◆ small quantity of plain flour
- ◆ 1 cup orange custard sauce (see
  recipe, page 174) or 1 cup
  (250ml) apple purée

⏱ 20 minutes

METHOD

1. Place milk and nutmeg in small saucepan and bring
   to boil.
2. Remove from heat and quickly stir in semolina.
3. Return to heat and stir for one minute.
4. Add egg, vanilla, peel, currants and sultanas and mix well.
5. Turn onto a lightly floured board and knead gently
   until smooth.
6. Break off small, even-sized pieces and roll into balls the
   size of large marbles. Toss each ball in flour.
7. Half fill a large saucepan with water and bring to boil.
8. Drop dumplings into boiling water and cook for approximately five minutes. (Note: the dumplings will rise to the
   top of the water as they cook.)
9. Drain and serve immediately with orange custard sauce
   or apple purée.

NUTRITION DATA PER SERVING:
140 kcal (584 kJ), CHO 24g, protein 7g, fat 2g.

BAKED YOGHURT SLICE

SERVES EIGHT

- 12 wheatmeal biscuits or 1 cup (130g) Meg's muesli (see recipe, page 56)
- 2–3 tablespoons unsweetened apple juice, for base
- 1 cup (250ml) low-fat fruit yoghurt
- 1¼ cups (325g) ricotta cheese
- juice of 1 lemon
- rind of 1 lemon, grated
- 2 tablespoons unsweetened apple juice, for filling
- 2 egg whites
- ½ cup (85g) sultanas

⏱ 1 hour

VARIATION: Use different flavoured yoghurt.

METHOD

1. Grind the biscuits or muesli in food processor or blender or crush well with rolling pin.
2. Add apple juice to biscuit crumbs to make a spreadable mixture.
3. Line tart tin with aluminium foil.
4. Press the biscuit crumb mixture into lined tart tin.
5. Blend yoghurt, ricotta cheese, lemon juice and rind and apple juice in food processor or blender.
6. Beat egg whites stiffly. Fold through the blended cheese mixture with the sultanas. Pour into biscuit base.
7. Bake in a preheated 180°C (350°F) oven for approximately 30 minutes until firm.
8. Cool and cut into slices.

NUTRITION DATA PER SERVING:
187 kcal (781 kJ), CHO 25g, protein 8g, fat 6g.

MOCHA MOUSSE

- 2 eggs, separated
- 1½ cups (375ml) evaporated milk
- 1 tablespoon cocoa
- ½ teaspoon instant coffee granules
- 3 teaspoons gelatine
- 3 tablespoons water
- 3 sachets Candarel™ artificial sweetener equivalent to 6 teaspoons sugar
- chopped dates or fresh strawberries, for garnish

⏱ 45 minutes, plus overnight setting time

This is a scrumptious dessert. Prepare it the day before you want to serve it because it needs to set.

METHOD

1. Beat egg yolks, and combine in a saucepan with milk, cocoa and coffee. Mix until smooth.
2. Stirring constantly, warm the mixture over medium heat, being careful not to boil. Remove from heat and cool.
3. Sprinkle gelatine over water and dissolve over hot water, or microwave on medium for 10 seconds. Cool slightly.
4. Stir into chocolate mixture. Add sweetener. Cool until mixture begins to set around edges.
5. Whip until thick and creamy.
6. Beat egg whites until soft peaks form. Fold into chocolate mixture.
7. Pour into serving dishes. Cover and refrigerate overnight.
8. Serve chilled and garnish with chopped dates or strawberries.

NUTRITION DATA PER SERVING:
184 kcal (768 kJ), CHO 16g, protein 17g, fat 14g.

BAKED CUSTARD

SERVES FOUR

- 2 eggs
- liquid artificial sweetener to taste
- 1⅓ cups (330ml) skimmed milk
- 1 teaspoon vanilla essence
- sprinkling of ground nutmeg

⏱ 1 hour 10 minutes

This family favourite can be served hot or cold.

METHOD

1. Lightly beat the eggs in a bowl.
2. Gradually add the milk to the egg mixture, stirring constantly. Stir in the vanilla essence and sweetener. Check flavour.
3. Pour mixture into a deep pie or soufflé dish or four single-serve oven-proof dishes. Sprinkle with nutmeg.
4. Stand the baking dish(es) in a large baking dish. Carefully pour enough water into the large baking dish to reach two-thirds up the outside of the pie or soufflé dish(es).
5. Bake in a preheated 150°C (300°F) oven for 35 minutes if you are using individual dishes, 45 minutes if you are using one big dish. The custard should be lightly browned and set in the centre.

NUTRITION DATA PER SERVING:
63 kcal (266 kJ), CHO 4g, protein 6g, fat 3g.

CRÊPES SUZETTE

SERVES FOUR

- 4 oranges, peeled and cut into segments, pith removed
- juice of 1 orange
- 3 tablespoons brandy
- 12 crêpes (see recipe, page 134), warmed
- rind of 1 orange, grated

⏱ 10 minutes

METHOD

1. Poach orange segments gently in orange juice until heated through.
2. Drain off juice and set aside.
3. Add brandy to fruit in frying pan, heat and ignite with a match or a lighter. Stir fruit gently and allow brandy to burn out.
4. Pour juice back into pan and reheat.
5. Place crêpes one by one in pan, filling each with fruit, and folding each into four to make a triangle. This allows crêpes to absorb the juice.
6. Serve topped with sprinkling of orange rind.

NUTRITION DATA PER SERVING:
237 kcal (992 kJ), CHO 37g, protein 10g, fat 5g.

BERRY AND CHEESE PANCAKES

SERVES FOUR

- 2 cups (300g) mixed berries, washed and hulled
- 1 teaspoon water
- 8 pancakes (see recipe, page 134), warmed
- 8 tablespoons cottage cheese

⏱ 5 minutes

METHOD

1. Poach berries in water for approximately three minutes until soft.
2. Divide fruit evenly between pancakes and top each with 1 tablespoon cottage cheese.
3. Roll up and serve hot.

NUTRITION DATA PER SERVING:
266 kcal (1158 kJ), CHO 29g, protein 16g, fat 9g.

BUCKWHEAT PANCAKES WITH BLUEBERRY SAUCE

SERVES FOUR (2 pancakes each)

- ½ cup (70g) buckwheat flour
- ½ cup (70g) plain flour
- 2 teaspoons baking powder
- ½ teaspoon cinnamon
- 1 tablespoon sugar
- 1 egg, beaten
- ¾ cup (190ml) semi-skimmed milk
- 1 quantity blueberry sauce (see recipe, page 173)

⏱ 30 minutes

METHOD

1. Sift flours, baking powder, and cinnamon into a mixing bowl. Return any husks to bowl.
2. Add sugar and mix in well.
3. Beat egg and milk together.
4. Stir egg mixture slowly into the centre of the flour mixture, bringing flour in from the sides as you mix, then beat well until there are no lumps.
5. Heat frying pan, spraying with a little baking spray to prevent sticking.
6. Spoon 2 tablespoons mixture into pan, cooking two pancakes at a time. When bubbles appear on the surface, turn the pancakes and cook on the other side until golden brown.
7. Keep warm until all pancakes are cooked.
8. Spoon over the blueberry sauce and serve.

NUTRITION DATA PER SERVING:
165 kcal (691 kJ), CHO 28g, protein 7.5g, fat 2.5g.

APPLE AND SULTANA PANCAKES

SERVES FOUR

- ◆ 4 apples, peeled, cored and sliced
- ◆ 2 cloves
- ◆ 2 tablespoons sultanas
- ◆ 8 pancakes (see recipe, page 134), warmed

⏱ 10 minutes

METHOD

1. Poach apples gently in a little water with cloves and sultanas for approximately five minutes until soft. Alternatively, microwave, covered, on high for five to eight minutes.
2. Remove cloves and divide apple mixture evenly between pancakes.
3. Roll up and serve hot.

NUTRITION DATA PER SERVING:
283 kcal (1183 kJ), CHO 50g, protein 10g, fat 5g.

GOLDEN FRUIT FLUMMERY

SERVES TWELVE

- ◆ 1 packet low-calorie jelly crystals, orange or orange and mango flavours
- ◆ 1½ cups (375ml) boiling water
- ◆ ½ cup (125ml) canned evaporated skimmed milk, chilled
- ◆ 400g can solid packed unsweetened peach pieces, puréed
- ◆ 1 large mango, puréed
- ◆ low-fat fruit yoghurt, to serve
- ◆ sprig of mint, for garnish

⏱ 2 hours

VARIATION: Purée one 400g can solid packed unsweetened apricot pieces instead of peaches and mango.

To prevent the evaporated milk separating from the rest of the flummery, you need to have the jelly and milk mixtures at approximately the same temperature before you combine them.

METHOD

1. Dissolve jelly crystals in boiling water, cool, place in refrigerator until just beginning to set.
2. Whip jelly and, as it becomes fluffy, slowly add evaporated skimmed milk, whipping continually until the mixture thickens.
3. Gently mix in puréed fruit and pour into glass dishes.
4. Chill well before serving, garnished with a spoonful of yoghurt and a sprig of mint on each dish.

NUTRITION DATA PER SERVING:
31 kcal (131 kJ), CHO 6g, protein 2g, fat trace.

BAKED APPLES WITH ORANGE AND STRAWBERRY SAUCE

SERVES FOUR

- ◆ 4 Granny Smith apples
- ◆ cinnamon
- ◆ 1 cup (250ml) orange juice
- ◆ 1 punnet strawberries
- ◆ liquid artificial sweetener to taste
- ◆ 2 tablespoons slivered almonds or chopped pecans
- ◆ orange slices

⏱ 1 hour

METHOD

1. Peel and core apples. When peeling, leave some peel on, to create a horizontal striped effect.
2. Place in a small baking dish. Sprinkle with cinnamon, then pour on the orange juice.
3. Bake, covered, in a preheated 180°C (350°F) oven for 30–35 minutes, or microwave on high for six to eight minutes, until the apples are tender but still retain their shape. Baste occasionally to prevent drying out.
4. While apples are cooking, wash, hull and purée strawberries. Add sweetener to purée.
5. When apples are cooked, lift gently onto individual serving dishes.
6. Reduce cooking liquid by boiling if necessary, and pour into strawberry purée. Mix and pour over apples.
7. Decorate with slivered nuts and orange slices.
8. Serve warm or chilled.

NUTRITION DATA PER SERVING:
92 kcal (387 kJ), CHO 18g, protein 2g, fat 1g.

ENGLISH FRUIT COMPOTE

SERVES FOUR

- 1 small apple, peeled, cored and cut into 8 wedges
- 1 cup unsweetened canned peaches in natural juice, made up of approximately ½ cup peaches and ½ cup (125ml) liquid
- 1 small pear, peeled, cored and cut into 8 wedges
- 12 whole cherries
- 4 yellow plums, cut into half and stoned
- 2 cloves
- pinch ground cinnamon

⏱ 2 hours 20 minutes

This is usually a chilled dessert, but you can serve it hot. Vary the fruit according to season and your preference. For instance, if fresh plums are not available, use canned, unsweetened apricot halves or peach slices which you add after the other fruit has been cooked.

METHOD

1. Place ingredients in a saucepan, with apple at the bottom and peaches on the top.
2. Bring to the boil and simmer gently for 10 minutes or until all fruit is tender. Alternatively, place fruit in a microwave dish, cover and cook on medium for five minutes.
3. Cool and place in refrigerator for at least two hours before serving in glass dishes.

NUTRITION DATA PER SERVING:
68 kcal (283 kJ), CHO 16g, protein 1g, fat 0g.

FLAMBÉED PANCAKES OR CRÊPES

SERVES FOUR

- 1 punnet strawberries, washed and hulled
- 2 bananas, sliced
- 8 apricots, stoned and quartered
- juice of 1 orange
- ½ teaspoon ground cinnamon
- 4 tablespoons brandy
- 8 pancakes or 12 crêpes (see recipe, page 134), warmed

⏱ 10 minutes

VARIATION: You can use any mixture of fruits.

METHOD

1. In a frying pan, combine fruit, orange juice and cinnamon and simmer gently for approximately five minutes until fruit heats through and softens.
2. Drain off juice and set aside.
3. Add brandy to pan, heat and ignite with a match or lighter, being careful not to burn yourself. Stir gently and allow brandy to burn out.
4. Pour juice back into pan and reheat.
5. Divide fruit evenly between pancakes or crêpes and roll up or, if using crêpes, fold into four to make triangles.

NUTRITION DATA PER SERVING:
296 kcal (1236 kJ), CHO 59g, protein 12g, fat 5g.

SUMMER PUDDING

SERVES FOUR

- 14 slices wholegrain bread, crusts removed
- 6 cups (900g) mixed fresh berries (strawberries, raspberries, blueberries, loganberries)
- 4 teaspoons caster sugar
- extra berries, for garnish

🕐 20 minutes, plus overnight refrigeration

METHOD

1. Cut crusts off bread and discard them.
2. Cut four round bases and tops out of bread. Set tops aside. Place a base in four individual soufflé dishes. Use the remaining bread to line the sides of the dishes. Do this carefully, making sure that there are no gaps.
3. Wash and hull berries. Chop strawberries.
4. Place berries and sugar in saucepan, and heat gently until liquid runs from berries.
5. Fill soufflé dishes, packing fruit down firmly, and pour over the juice.
6. Cover each with one of the reserved tops.
7. Place a weight on top and refrigerate overnight.
8. Remove and discard the tops.
9. Turn onto serving dishes. Garnish with extra berries.

NUTRITION DATA PER SERVING:
209 kcal (876 kJ), CHO 42g, protein 7g, fat 1g.

GINGER PEARS

SERVES FOUR

- 4 medium pears, peeled and quartered
- 285ml bottle low-calorie dry ginger ale
- juice of 1 lemon
- ½ teaspoon minced fresh ginger
- ¼ cup (60ml) orange juice concentrate
- 3–4 drops yellow food colouring (optional)
- 6 cloves
- ground cinnamon, for garnish

🕐 1 hour

METHOD

1. Place pears in a saucepan. Add dry ginger ale, lemon juice, ginger, orange juice concentrate, food colouring and cloves.
2. Cover and simmer until pears are tender, turning and basting the pears so they cook and colour evenly Alternatively, microwave, covered, on high for four to six minutes until tender.
3. Lift pears onto serving dish.
4. Simmer juice until slightly reduced.
5. Pour over pears. Sprinkle with cinnamon.
6. Serve hot or chilled.

NUTRITION DATA PER SERVING:
91 kcal (382 kJ), CHO 22g, protein 1g, fat 0g.

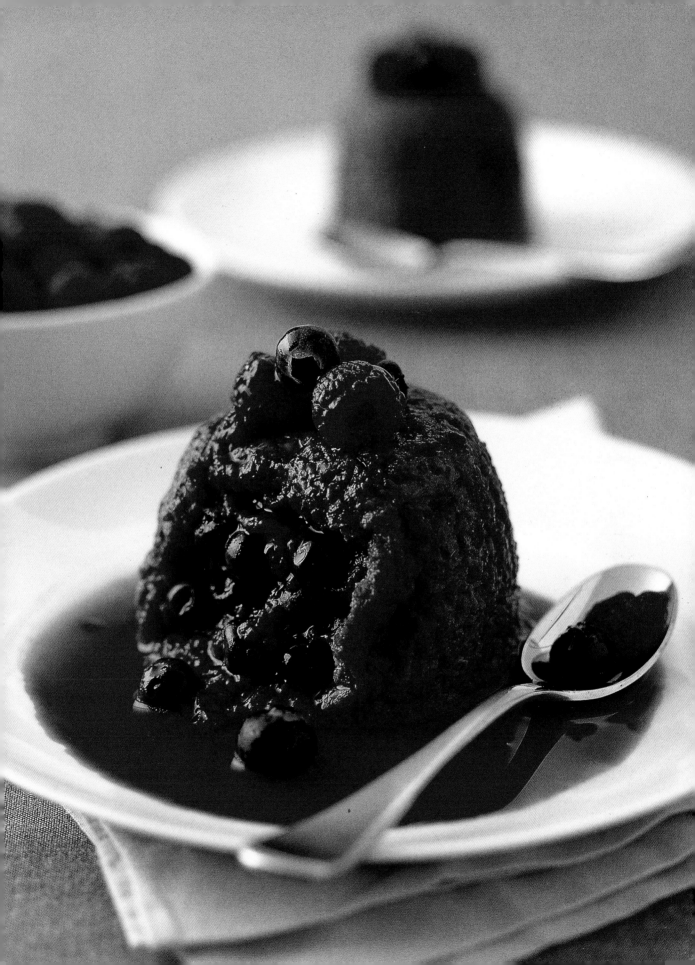

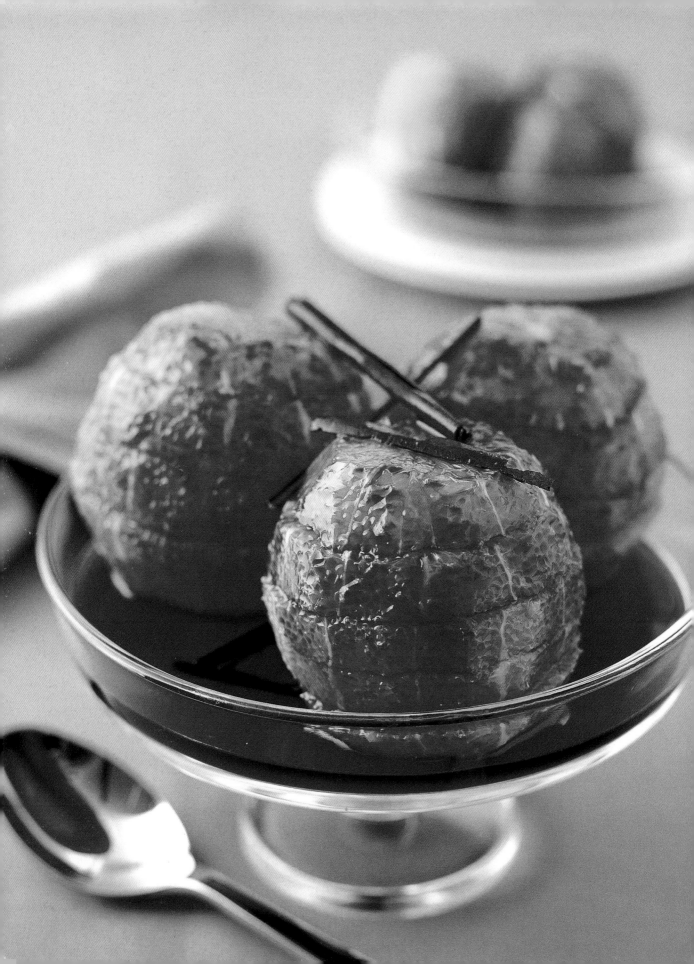

SPICED ORANGES

SERVES SIX

- 2 cups (500ml) red wine, such as claret or burgundy
- 1 cup (250ml) unsweetened orange juice
- ½ teaspoon ground cinnamon or 2 cinnamon sticks
- 6 oranges
- Candarel™ or other artificial sweetener to taste

⏱ 15 minutes

The ideal dessert after a long hot summer's day.

METHOD
1. Place wine, orange juice and cinnamon in a saucepan and bring to the boil.
2. Boil hard for two minutes, then remove from heat, or microwave on high for two to three minutes.
3. Peel oranges, removing all pith, slice horizontally and arrange in a glass serving bowl.
4. Pour wine mixture over oranges.
5. Chill well and sweeten before serving.

NUTRITION DATA PER SERVING:
52 kcal (219 kJ), CHO 11g, protein 1g, fat trace.

CREAMY RICE

SERVES FOUR

- 1 cup (200g) basmati rice
- 1½ cups (375ml) water
- 2½ cups (600ml) skimmed or semi-skimmed milk
- ½ cup (85g) sultanas
- ½ teaspoon ground nutmeg
- 1 teaspoon vanilla essence
- 2 sachets of Candarel™ or artificial sweetener equivalent to 4 teaspoons sugar

⏱ 1 hour

METHOD
1. Wash rice and place in saucepan, cover with the water, and simmer over very low heat until water is absorbed.
2. Add 1 cup milk. Simmer again until absorbed.
3. Add the remaining 1½ cups milk and cook again until the milk is absorbed.
4. Stir in sultanas, nutmeg, vanilla and sweetener to taste.
5. Serve warm with sliced stewed or fresh fruit.

NUTRITION DATA PER SERVING:
283 kcal (1185 kJ), CHO 58 g, protein 10g, fat 1g.

LEMON AND CINNAMON CHEESECAKE

SERVES EIGHT

- 1 cup (130g) wheatmeal biscuit crumbs
- 50g ground almonds or almond meal
- 1 tablespoon margarine, melted
- 2 teaspoons water
- 2 teaspoons cinnamon
- 1¼ cups (300ml) buttermilk
- 250g ricotta cheese
- juice of 2 lemons
- rind of 1 lemon, grated
- 1 teaspoon vanilla essence
- 1 tablespoon sugar, or Candarel™, or other equivalent artificial sweetener
- 1 tablespoon powdered gelatine
- 2 tablespoons water
- kiwifruit and/or strawberries, for garnish
- 2 teaspoons cinnamon, for garnish

⏱ 1 hour

VARIATION: Replace lemons and lemon rind with the juice and rind of 1 orange.

You must make this recipe the day before you want to serve it to allow the filling to set.

METHOD

1. Combine biscuit crumbs, ground almonds, margarine, water and cinnamon.
2. Press mixture into a lined 20cm springform cake tin and refrigerate for 30 minutes.
3. Mix buttermilk with ricotta cheese, lemon juice, lemon rind, vanilla essence and sugar or artificial sweetener. Beat until smooth and fluffy.
4. Dissolve gelatine in hot water. Cool slightly, fold into buttermilk mixture and blend well.
5. Pour into pie dish and refrigerate until set.
6. Next day, decorate with sliced kiwifruit and a sprinkle of cinnamon.

NUTRITION DATA PER SERVING:
191 kcal (800 kJ), CHO 14g, protein 7g, fat 12g.

CREAMY BAKED CHEESECAKE

SERVES EIGHT

- 125g wheatmeal biscuits, crushed
- 1 tablespoon ground almonds or almond meal
- 60g poly- or monounsaturated margarine
- 250g ricotta cheese
- 100g plain cottage cheese
- 1 tablespoon fine semolina
- 100g low-fat fruit yoghurt
- ¼–½ cup (50–100g) caster sugar
- 3 eggs, separated
- 1 teaspoon grated lemon rind
- 2 teaspoons lemon juice
- 1 cup (290g) fruit pulp (e.g. mango, berries, apricots or other fruit) or ½ cup (120g) passionfruit pulp

⏱ 1 hour 30 minutes

METHOD

1. Combine biscuit crumbs, ground almonds and margarine. Spread over the base of a lightly greased 20cm springform cake tin and set aside.
2. Place ricotta cheese, cottage cheese, semolina, yoghurt, sugar and egg yolks in a food processor or blender and process until smooth.
3. Beat egg whites until soft peaks form.
4. Fold cheese mixture into egg whites, then lightly fold through lemon rind and fruit. Spoon mixture into prepared tin and bake at 180°C (350°F) for 50–55 minutes or until firm. Cool in pan.

NUTRITION DATA PER SERVING:
241 kcal (1008 kJ), CHO 17g, protein 11g, fat 15g.

RICOTTA RAISIN FLAN

SERVES SIX TO EIGHT

- 2 tablespoons margarine
- 125g wheatmeal biscuits, crushed
- 500g ricotta cheese
- 4 tablespoons apple concentrate
- 1 cup (160g) raisins, chopped
- rind of 1 lemon, grated
- ½ teaspoon ground cinnamon
- ¼ teaspoon ground nutmeg
- 1 egg
- ½ cup (125ml) semi-skimmed milk

⏱ 1 hour 50 minutes

METHOD

1. Melt margarine, then pour onto biscuit crumbs and mix.
2. Spread over base and up sides of pie dish. Press well to make an even, firm crust.
3. Bake in a preheated 180°C (350°F) oven for 10 minutes. Cool.
4. Mix ricotta, apple concentrate, raisins, lemon rind and spices.
5. Beat egg and combine with milk. Mix it with other ingredients. Blend well.
6. Pour into pie dish. Bake for 30–45 minutes until set and lightly browned.
7. Sprinkle with a little cinnamon and serve.

NUTRITION DATA PER SERVING:
373 kcal (1562 kJ), CHO 43 g, protein 13g, fat 17g.

LEMON DELICIOUS

SERVES FOUR

- 3 eggs
- 5 tablespoons fresh lemon juice
- rind of 1 lemon, grated
- 1 tablespoon melted butter
- 3 tablespoons wholemeal plain flour
- 1½ cups (375ml) semi-skimmed milk
- 1 tablespoon sugar or equivalent in artificial sweetener

⏱ 1 hour

METHOD

1. Separate eggs. Beat egg whites until stiff peaks form.
2. Beat yolks with the remaining ingredients until smooth.
3. Gradually fold the egg whites into mixture.
4. Spoon evenly into four dishes.
5. Place in a larger baking dish. Carefully pour water into the larger baking dish until it reaches two-thirds up the outside of the individual baking dishes.
6. Bake in a preheated 160°C (325°F) oven for approximately 20 minutes or until set and lightly browned.
7. Cool slightly in the water-filled dish to prevent shrinking.

NUTRITION DATA PER SERVING:
212 kcal (886 kJ), CHO 12g, protein 9g, fat 14g.

CRUNCHY PEACH ICE CREAM

SERVES SIX TO EIGHT

- 425g can solid-pack pie peaches
- juice of ½ lemon
- ½ teaspoon ground cinnamon
- 50g ricotta cheese
- 100g low-fat natural yoghurt
- Candarel™ or 2 tablespoons apple concentrate to taste
- 2 teaspoons liqueur (optional)
- 2 tablespoons dessicated coconut
- 2 tablespoons chopped blanched almonds, toasted
- 3 tablespoons crunchy cereal (e.g. muesli, rice krispies, etc.)
- 1 egg white

⏱ 1 hour plus freezing time

The more carefully you beat the mixture part way through the freezing process, the smoother and creamier your ice cream will be. Homemade ice cream is better used fresh as it tends to go hard if refrozen.

METHOD
1. Blend fruit in food processor or blender until smooth and creamy.
2. Add other ingredients and blend well. Add liqueur if desired.
3. Spoon into a container with a lid. Cover and freeze for two to three hours until almost set.
4. Remove and thaw slightly. Break up the ice crystals by returning to food processor or blender, blend until creamy, then spoon back into bowl and add coconut, nuts and cereal.
5. Beat egg white until soft peaks form.
6. Fold into ice cream, cover and refreeze until firm.
7. Remove and allow to thaw a little before serving as this ice cream is much more delicious if eaten a little soft.

NUTRITION DATA PER SERVING:
83 kcal (348 kJ), CHO 7g, protein 4g, fat 4g.

BREAD AND BUTTER PUDDING

SERVES FOUR

- 4 eggs
- 2½ cups (600ml) skimmed or semi-skimmed milk
- 2 teaspoons vanilla essence
- 3 slices wholegrain bread
- 2 teaspoons margarine
- 2 tablespoons sultanas
- 1 teaspoon ground nutmeg

⏱ 1 hour

METHOD

1. Place eggs in bowl and beat.
2. Add milk and vanilla essence.
3. Spread bread with margarine and cut each slice into four squares.
4. Place three squares in each of four individual baking dishes.
5. Pour an equal amount of the mixture into each dish.
6. Sprinkle sultanas and nutmeg evenly into the four dishes.
7. Place the four individual dishes in a larger baking dish, and carefully pour water into the larger baking dish to reach two-thirds up the outside of the individual baking dishes.
8. Bake in a preheated 180°C (350°F) oven for 30–45 minutes until set, or arrange the puddings in a wide circle in the microwave to ensure even cooking. Microwave on medium for 8–10 minutes.

NUTRITION DATA PER SERVING:
200 kcal (837 kJ), CHO 19g, protein 13g, fat 8g.

QUEEN'S PUDDING

SERVES FOUR

- ◆ 4 eggs
- ◆ 2½ cups (600ml) skimmed or semi-skimmed milk
- ◆ 2 teaspoons vanilla essence
- ◆ 3 slices wholegrain bread, crumbed
- ◆ 4 tablespoons strawberry or raspberry purée
- ◆ 1 tablespoon caster sugar

⏱ 1 hour 30 minutes

If you do not have any strawberry or raspberry purée, you can use reduced-sugar jam as a substitute.

METHOD

1. Separate two eggs and put egg whites aside.
2. Combine egg yolks with the other two whole eggs and beat.
3. Add milk and vanilla.
4. Distribute breadcrumbs evenly between four individual baking dishes.
5. Pour equal amounts of custard mixture into each dish.
6. Put individual dishes in a larger baking dish, and carefully pour in water until it reaches two-thirds up the outside of the individual baking dishes. Bake in a preheated 180°C (350°F) oven for 30–45 minutes.
7. When cooked, carefully spread top of custard with fruit purée.
8. Beat the remaining two egg whites until they are stiff and fold in caster sugar and pile over purée.
9. Bake for about five minutes until meringue is lightly browned.

NUTRITION DATA PER SERVING:
189 kcal (793 kJ), CHO 21g, protein 13g, fat 6g.

CHRISTMAS PUDDING

SERVES SIX

- ◆ 4 tablespoons sultanas
- ◆ 2 tablespoons currants
- ◆ 3 tablespoons raisins
- ◆ rind of 1 orange, grated
- ◆ ½ cup (70g) grated carrot, apple or cooked pumpkin (or a mixture of any two)
- ◆ 3 tablespoons brandy
- ◆ ½ cup (70g) wholemeal flour
- ◆ 1 teaspoon ground cinnamon
- ◆ 1 teaspoon mixed spice
- ◆ ½ teaspoon nutmeg
- ◆ 2 tablespoons margarine
- ◆ 1½ slices wholegrain bread, crumbed
- ◆ 1 egg, lightly beaten
- ◆ ⅓ cup (80ml) skimmed or semi-skimmed milk
- ◆ 1 teaspoon vanilla essence
- ◆ 1 tablespoon brown sugar
- ◆ ½ teaspoon bicarbonate of soda
- ◆ 1 tablespoon hot water

🕐 2 hours 20 minutes
plus overnight soaking

This is better made a week before you want to serve it, to allow the flavours time to mature.

METHOD

1. Soak dried fruit, orange rind and carrot, apple or pumpkin in brandy overnight.
2. Mix flour and spices.
3. Rub margarine into flour mixture, and add breadcrumbs.
4. Add egg, milk, fruit mixture, vanilla, and sugar or sweetener.
5. Combine bicarbonate of soda and hot water and mix well with other ingredients.
6. Pour into a greased bowl or pudding basin, cover securely and steam for 1½–2 hours.
7. Turn out and serve with brandy sauce (see recipe, page 174).

NUTRITION DATA PER SERVING:
298 kcal (1246 kJ), CHO 46g, protein 10g, fat 6g.

BAKING

By tradition, many baked products, especially pastries, cakes and biscuits, are high in fat, sugar and additives and low in fibre and other nutrients. These days, however, the trend is often towards healthier foods and some good breads, cakes and biscuits are now available commercially. In this section we have included a range of products—muffins that can make excellent breakfasts, lunches or snacks and cakes and biscuits that can be part of your regular meal plan or used for a more special occasion.

In our recipes we frequently use wholemeal flours which add fibre and other nutrients. When replacing white flours with wholemeal flours in cooking, slightly more fluid is needed to prevent the finished product being too dry. If you are hesitant about substituting wholemeal for white flour in a favourite recipe, begin by using half wholemeal and half white flour. As you see how successful this can be, you will soon gain confidence to use a greater proportion of the wholemeal flour.

Fresh home baked bread is wonderful. Try the quick wholemeal bread (see recipe, page 203) which is yeast free and therefore requires no rising time. Nor does it require kneading which adds to its simplicity. If you are used to baking your own bread, try adding grains such as barley, oats and rice bran to your bread mix. This helps lower the glycaemic index and is a good way to improve nutrition at a low cost.

HERBY CORN MUFFINS

MAKES TWELVE

- ◆ 1 cup (140g) plain flour
- ◆ 1 cup (130g) cornmeal
- ◆ ½ teaspoon salt
- ◆ 2 teaspoons baking powder
- ◆ 1 tablespoon margarine, melted
- ◆ 1 cup (250ml) semi-skimmed milk
- ◆ 1 egg, beaten
- ◆ ¼ teaspoon black pepper
- ◆ ½ teaspoon dried mixed herbs
- ◆ 2 tablespoons grated reduced-fat cheddar cheese

🕐 30 minutes

These savoury muffins are a great accompaniment to pumpkin or corn chowder. Eat them fresh because they won't keep.

METHOD

1. Sift flours, salt and baking powder into a bowl.
2. Mix margarine, milk and egg and add to dry ingredients. Beat until smooth.
3. Fold in seasonings and cheese and spoon mixture into lightly greased muffin tins.
4. Bake in a preheated 210°C (425°F) oven for 15–20 minutes until golden brown. Turn out to cool.

NUTRITION DATA PER MUFFIN:
112 kcal (471 kJ), CHO 17g, protein 4g, fat 3g.

WHOLEMEAL DAMPER

SERVES SIX

- ◆ 2 cups (280g) wholemeal self-raising flour
- ◆ ¼ teaspoon salt
- ◆ 2 teaspoons margarine
- ◆ ⅓ cup (80ml) skimmed or semi-skimmed milk
- ◆ ⅔ cup (160ml) water
- ◆ 1 tablespoon sesame seeds

🕐 50 minutes

METHOD

1. Sift flour and salt into mixing bowl. Return bran to sifted flour.
2. Rub margarine into flour until mixture resembles fine breadcrumbs.
3. Combine milk and water, and pour into dry ingredients. Mix quickly, blending with a knife.
4. Turn onto a floured board. Work into a round shape.
5. Place on lightly greased baking tray. Sprinkle with sesame seeds. Bake in a preheated 220°C (440°F) oven for 20–30 minutes until brown. Eat while warm.

NUTRITION DATA PER SERVING:
183 kcal (767 kJ), CHO 31g, protein 7g, fat 3g.

BANANA MUFFINS

MAKES TWELVE

- 2 very ripe bananas
- 1 egg
- ½ cup (125ml) skimmed or semi-skimmed milk
- ½ cup (125ml) unsweetened apple juice
- 1 cup (140g) wholemeal self-raising flour
- 1 cup (140g) white self-raising flour
- ½ teaspoon ground cinnamon
- ½ teaspoon baking powder

⏱ 40 minutes

Muffins for breakfast, muffins for school lunch, muffins as a snack…muffins are full of carbohydrate and fibre.

METHOD

1. Mash bananas very well. There should be no lumps.
2. Beat egg and add to banana.
3. Add milk and apple juice.
4. Sift flours, cinnamon and baking powder.
5. Fold flours into liquid mixture. Mix well, by hand.
6. Spoon into very lightly greased muffin tins, filling each up by about two thirds.
7. Bake in a preheated 210°C (425°F) oven for about 20 minutes until lightly browned and cooked through.
8. Remove from oven, lift muffins out of tins and cool on a cake rack.

NUTRITION DATA PER MUFFIN:
112 kcal (468 kJ), CHO 21g, protein 4g, fat 1g.

CHRIS' COOKIES

MAKES TWENTY-FOUR COOKIES

- 1 cup (100g) rolled oats
- 1 cup (140g) wholemeal self-raising flour
- ½ cup (70g) rice bran or oat bran
- ½ cup (70g) Candarel™ (or equivalent granulated sweetener)
- ½ cup (40g) desiccated coconut
- ½ cup (80g) currants
- 2 large very ripe bananas, mashed
- 2 eggs, beaten

⏱ 25 minutes

You can use sultanas or chopped dried apricots instead of currants to make these quick and easy cookies.

METHOD

1. Mix dry ingredients, add banana and eggs and mix well.
2. Break off small pieces and roll into balls. Place on lightly greased oven trays and flatten each ball with the back of a fork.
3. Bake in a preheated 180°C (350°F) oven for about 15 minutes or until just beginning to brown.
4. Remove from oven trays, and cool on a cake rack.

NUTRITION DATA PER COOKIE:
117 kcal (489 kJ), CHO 18g, protein 4g, fat 3g.

WHOLEMEAL PASTRY

- 1 cup (140g) wholemeal flour
- 1 cup (140g) plain flour
- 120g margarine
- juice of ½ lemon
- ½–¾ cup (125ml–190ml) iced water

⏱ 15 minutes

You can use 2 cups of wholemeal flour if you like, but the pastry will be heavier than the version we suggest here. A food processor is a great help; it turns pastry-making into a quick and easy process, but be careful not to over-process the pastry or it will become heavy.

METHOD
1. Combine the flours in a large bowl.
2. Rub the margarine into the flour until the mixture resembles breadcrumbs.
3. Combine juice and water and add it to the dry ingredients, a little at a time, working it in after each addition, until you have a soft dough.
4. Turn dough onto a lightly floured board and knead lightly. Cover and allow to rest before using.
5. Use dough as required.

NOTE: Most pastries need to be baked in a hot oven—200°C (400°F)—for 15 minutes, or until lightly browned.

NUTRITION DATA PER QUANTITY:
1871 kcal (7831 kJ), CHO 193g, protein 36g, fat 104g.

PIKELETS

MAKES TWELVE TO SIXTEEN

- ¾ cup (95g) white self-raising flour
- ¾ cup (95g) wholemeal
  self-raising flour
- 1 egg
- ¾ cup (190ml) skimmed or
  semi-skimmed milk
- a little oil for frying

⏱ 30 minutes

We have given special recipes for conserves and spreads in this book; they are perfect served with these pikelets.

METHOD

1. Place flour in a basin and make a well in the centre.
2. Beat egg and mix in milk in a small bowl.
3. Pour the egg and milk mixture into the centre of the flour and gradually beat in the flour using a wooden spoon. Beat mixture well.
4. Heat frying pan and lightly oil.
5. Drop spoonfuls of mixture into pan allowing room for each pikelet to spread.
6. When mixture begins to bubble, turn over with a knife or egg slice.
7. Let pikelets cook until light brown on each side and lift onto a clean cloth. Keep covered with cloth to keep them soft.
8. Serve with dried apricot conserve (see recipe, page 58) or date and fig spread (see recipe, page 57).

NUTRITION DATA PER PIKELET:
81 kcal (341 kJ), CHO 13g, protein 3g, fat 2g.

BLUESTONE MUFFINS

MAKES TWELVE

- 1 cup (160g) ripe blueberries
- 4 teaspoons brown sugar
- 1 cup (140g) wholemeal
  self-raising flour
- 1 cup (140g) white self-raising flour
- 1 teaspoon baking powder
- 1 teaspoon ground cinnamon
- 1 egg
- ½ cup (125ml) low-fat
  berry yoghurt
- 1 cup (250ml) skimmed or
  semi-skimmed milk

⏱ 40 minutes

These muffins look a little strange, perhaps, but taste terrific. Eat them fresh; they won't keep. Remember, a trace of sugar will not harm you, particularly when combined with plenty of complex carbohydrate and fibre.

METHOD
1. Lightly grease muffin tins or spray with cooking spray.
2. Wash blueberries and combine with sugar in a saucepan.
3. Heat gently until juice just starts to run.
4. Sift flour, baking powder and cinnamon into a bowl. Return bran to flour mixture.
5. Mix egg, yoghurt and milk in a bowl. Add to flour and blend until smooth.
6. Gently fold blueberries into mixture.
7. Spoon mixture into muffin tins, and bake in a preheated 210°C (425°F) oven for 15–20 minutes until firm and very lightly browned.

NUTRITION DATA PER MUFFIN:
116 kcal (486 kJ), CHO 21g, protein 5g, fat 1g.

APPLE AND APRICOT SLICE

MAKES SIXTEEN SLICES

- 1 quantity wholemeal pastry (see recipe, page 200)
- 500g fresh apricots, stoned and quartered or 400g can unsweetened apricot pieces, drained
- 3 apples, peeled, cored and thinly sliced
- ½ teaspoon cinnamon
- skimmed milk for glazing

⏱ 50 minutes

METHOD
1. Divide pastry into two equal pieces. Roll out first half and cover base of lightly greased 28cm x 19cm biscuit tray.
2. Mix fruit and cinnamon and spread evenly on pastry.
3. Roll second half of pastry and place over fruit.
4. Prick surface of pastry with fork or skewer, brush with milk and bake in a preheated 200°C (400°F) oven for 30 minutes or until pastry is beginning to brown.
5. Stand on cake rack for five minutes, loosen around the edges and turn out. Cool and cut into 16 even pieces.

NUTRITION DATA PER PIECE:
136 kcal (569 kJ), CHO 17g, protein 3g, fat 7g.

QUICK WHOLEMEAL BREAD

MAKES TWO LOAVES

- 4 cups (560g) wholemeal flour
- 2 teaspoons bicarbonate of soda
- 2 cups (500 ml) wholemilk natural yoghurt
- 1 tablespoon honey (optional)
- 1 tablespoon sesame seeds (optional)

⏱ 1 hour

VARIATION: Add ½ cup (60g) roughly chopped pecan nuts or walnuts. Alternatively, try adding ½ cup (100g) sunflower seeds or raisins.

This quick and easy loaf contains no yeast, so there is no kneading and rising time required. You may prefer the flavour of the loaf with the addition of a little salt at step three, but try it without first.

METHOD
1. Lightly grease the loaf tin.
2. Measure the flour, unsifted, into a large bowl.
3. Add all remaining ingredients, except the sesame seeds. Use a wooden spoon to mix lightly but well, until mixture is fluffy.
4. Spoon mixture into the greased loaf tin. Sprinkle with sesame seeds.
5. Bake in a preheated 180°C (350°F) oven for 50–60 minutes, or until loaf sounds hollow when tapped.

NUTRITION DATA PER SLICE:
67 kcal (280 kJ), CHO 11g, protein 3g, fat 1g.

CARROT CAKE

MAKES TWENTY SLICES

- 2 cups (280g) wholemeal self-raising flour
- ½ teaspoon bicarbonate of soda
- 2 teaspoons ground cinnamon
- 1 teaspoon ground nutmeg
- 1 teaspoon mixed spice
- 2 cups (270g) grated carrot
- ½ cups (40g) dessicated coconut
- ½ cup (60g) chopped walnuts
- ½ cup (85g) sultanas
- 2 eggs
- ¼ cup (60ml) apple concentrate
- 1 cup (250ml) skimmed or semi-skimmed milk

⏱ 1 hour

METHOD

1. Grease and lightly flour a cake tin.
2. Sift flour, soda and spices. Return bran to flour mixture.
3. Add carrot, coconut, nuts and sultanas.
4. Beat eggs until fluffy and add apple concentrate. Beat again and add milk.
5. Fold into dry ingredients. Stir until well mixed and pour batter into a prepared 20cm cake tin.
6. Bake in a preheated 200°C (400°F) oven until cooked through (approximately 40–45 minutes).
7. Turn out and cool on a cake rack.

NUTRITION DATA PER SLICE:

113 kcal (475 kJ), CHO 16g, protein 4g, fat 4g.

DATE AND WALNUT LOAF

MAKES TEN SLICES

- ½ cup (125ml) boiling water
- 1 cup chopped dates
- 1½ cups wholemeal self-raising flour
- 1 teaspoon mixed spice
- 1 teaspoon ground cinnamon
- 2 tablespoons margarine
- 1 tablespoon sugar
- ½ cup chopped walnuts
- 1 egg, beaten
- 1 cup (250ml) skimmed milk

⏱ 1 hour 10 minutes

VARIATION: Replace dates and walnuts with any dried fruit of your choice.

METHOD

1. Pour boiling water over dates and let stand for 30 minutes.
2. Mix flour and spices in bowl.
3. Rub in margarine until mixture resembles breadcrumbs.
4. Add sugar, dates, soaking water and walnuts to dry mixture and mix lightly.
5. Stir in egg and skimmed milk.
6. Place in lightly greased loaf tin.
7. Bake in a preheated 190°C (375°F) oven for 20 minutes, then lower heat to 180°C (350°F) and bake for a further 25 minutes or until cooked.
8. Leave in tin for 10 minutes before turning out to cool.

NUTRITION DATA PER SLICE:

233 kcal (976 kJ), CHO 35g, protein 6g, fat 8g.

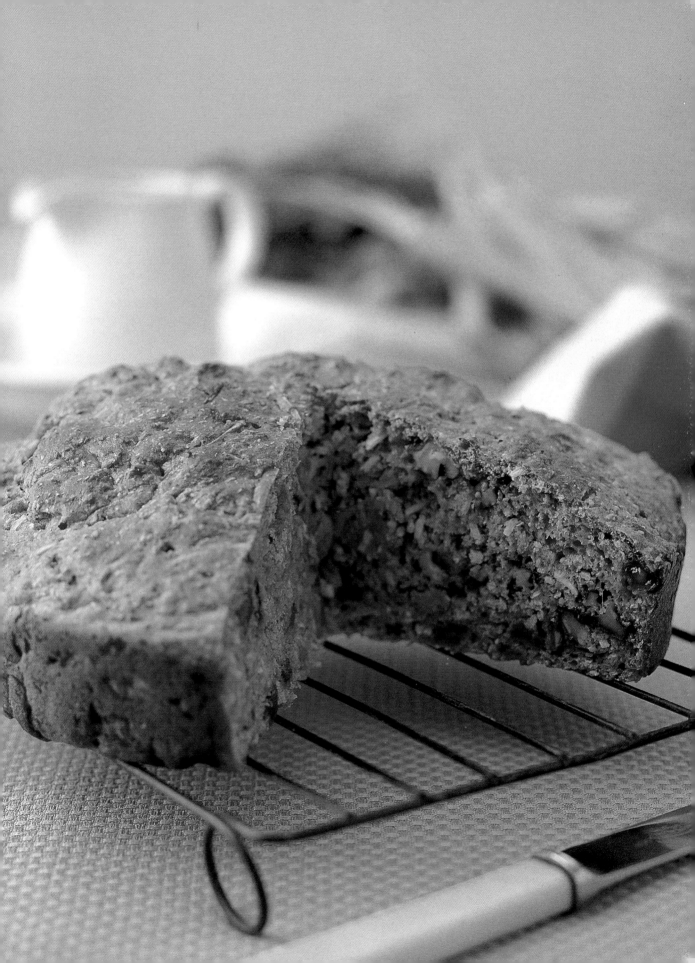

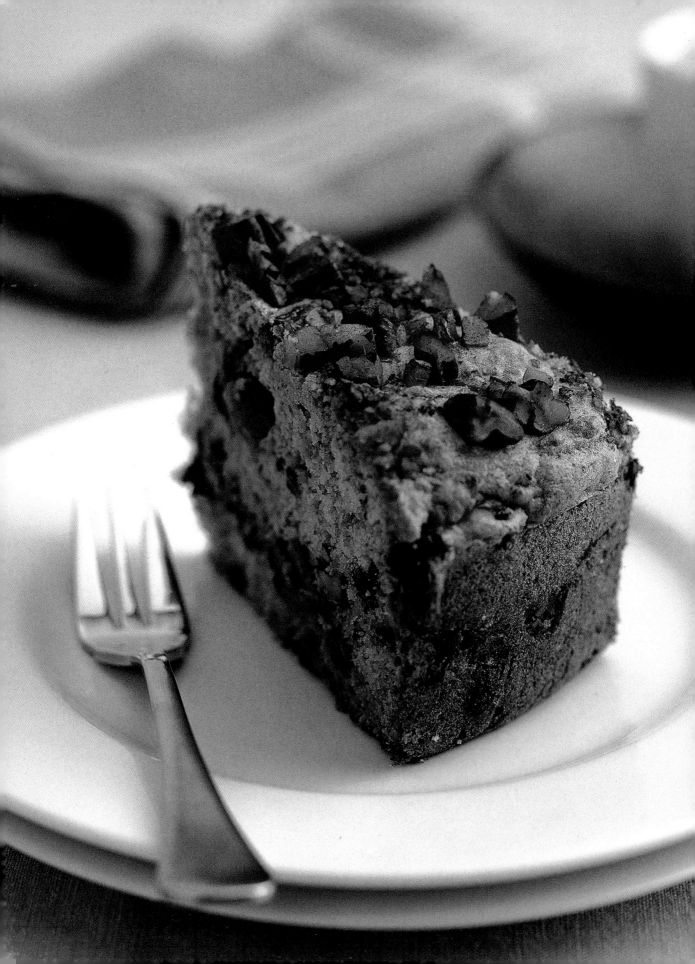

WHOLEMEAL APPLE–NUT STREUSEL CAKE

MAKES SIXTEEN SLICES

- 150g margarine
- ¾ cup Candarel™, or equivalent granulated sweetener
- 100g ricotta cheese
- 1 teaspoon vanilla essence
- 3 eggs
- ½ cup (70g) white self-raising flour
- 1½ cups (210g) wholemeal plain flour
- 1 teaspoon bicarbonate of soda
- 1 cup (250ml) skimmed milk
- 1 apple, peeled and grated
- ¾ cup (130g) sultanas
- 1 cup (130g) chopped pecans or walnuts
- ½ teaspoon ground cinnamon

⏱ 1 hour 15 minutes

METHOD

1. Lightly grease and line the base of a 20cm cake tin.
2. Cream margarine and Candarel™, then beat in ricotta and essence.
3. Add eggs one at a time and beat in.
4. Mix flours and soda and fold into mixture with milk.
5. Add apple and sultanas and mix.
6. Spread half the mixture into the cake tin. Sprinkle over half the nuts and cinnamon. Spread with remaining cake mixture and sprinkle with remaining nuts and cinnamon.
7. Bake in a preheated 180°C (350°F) oven for one hour or until cooked.
8. Cool slightly before turning out.

NUTRITION DATA PER SLICE:
193 kcal (807 kJ), CHO 15g, protein 5g, fat 13g.

FRUIT LOAF

MAKES SIXTEEN SLICES

- ½ cup (70g) chopped dried apricots
- ½ cup (80g) raisins
- ½ cup (65g) chopped walnuts
- 2 tablespoons margarine
- ⅓ cup powdered artificial sweetener suitable for baking
- 1 teaspoon mixed spice
- 1 teaspoon cinnamon
- 1 cup (250ml) hot water
- 1½ cups (210g) self-raising flour
- 1 teaspoon bicarbonate of soda
- ½ cup (125ml) semi-skimmed milk

⏱ 45 minutes

METHOD

1. Spray a loaf tin with spray oil.
2. Combine the apricots, raisins, walnuts, margarine, sweetener and spices in a mixing bowl and pour over the water.
3. Sift the self-raising flour and bicarbonate of soda together and fold into the fruit mixture.
4. Add the milk and fold in gently.
5. Spoon the mixture into the loaf tin and bake in a preheated 200°C (400°F) oven until brown and cooked through when tested with a skewer.
6. Turn out and cool before serving.

NUTRITION DATA PER SLICE:
113 kcal (474 kJ), CHO 15g, protein 3g, fat 5g.

MINCE TARTS

MAKES TWELVE

- ½ cup (70g) chopped dried apricots
- 1 cup (170g) sultanas
- ½ cup (90g) chopped pitted dates
- 12 prunes, seeded and chopped
- 6 dried figs, chopped
- ½ cup (70g) slivered almonds
- 2 apples, peeled, cored and thinly sliced
- ½ cup (125ml) brandy
- juice of ½ lemon
- ½ teaspoon cinnamon
- ½ teaspoon ground nutmeg
- ½ teaspoon mixed spice
- ½ cup (70g) wholemeal flour
- 1 cup (140g) plain flour
- 4 tablespoons margarine
- 2–3 tablespoons iced water
- 1 egg yolk
- few drops liquid artificial sweetener

🕐 1 hour 30 minutes plus overnight soaking

METHOD

1. Combine the fruits, almonds, brandy, lemon juice and spices in a saucepan.
2. Cook, covered, over low heat until apple is soft. Stir frequently to prevent sticking.
3. Spoon into a bowl, cover and refrigerate overnight to blend flavours.
4. Sift flours into another bowl, return bran left in sieve to sifted flour.
5. Rub margarine into flour until mixture resembles breadcrumbs.
6. In a cup combine water, egg yolk and sweetener.
7. Add to flour mixture and stir in with a knife. Turn out onto floured board. Knead lightly, then cover and leave to rest for 10–15 minutes.
8. Roll out dough and cut 12 rounds to fit the bottom of the tart tins. Cut another 12, slightly smaller, to make the lids.
9. Lightly grease the tart tins and line the bases with the pastry rounds.
10. Spoon some fruit mince into each.
11. Wet pastry edges and place remaining pastry rounds on top. Pinch edges to seal. Prick tops with fork.
12. Bake in a preheated 190°C (375°F) oven for 20–30 minutes until lightly browned.

NUTRITION DATA PER TART:
270 kcal (1130 kJ), CHO 43g, protein 5g, fat 9g.

FRUIT CAKE

- 1½ cups (255g) sultanas
- ½ cup (85g) raisins, chopped
- 2 tablespoons brandy
- 1 tablespoon water
- 1 cup (170g) sieved pumpkin (no lumps)
- 2 eggs, beaten
- ½ cup (125ml) apple concentrate
- ½ cup (125ml) skimmed or semi-skimmed milk
- ½ cup (60g) chopped pecans
- 1 teaspoon ground cinnamon
- 1 teaspoon mixed spice
- 1 cup (140g) white self-raising flour
- 1 cup (140g) wholemeal self-raising flour
- ½ teaspoon bicarbonate of soda

⏱ 1 hour 30 minutes plus overnight soaking

Apple concentrate gives sweetness to this wonderful fruity cake, and the dried fruit and pumpkin add plenty of fibre. It's perfect for Christmas.

METHOD

1. Mix sultanas, raisins, brandy and water. Leave to soak overnight.
2. Mix pumpkin, eggs, apple concentrate and milk.
3. Add soaked fruit, nuts and spices, then sifted flour and bicarbonate of soda. Return bran left in sieve to flour mixture. Mix well with a wooden spoon.
4. Spoon into a lightly greased round or square 20cm cake tin.
5. Bake for 10 minutes at 200°C (400°F), then turn down the heat and bake at 180°C (350°F) until cooked through and browned (approximately 1–1¼ hours). Cool on a cake rack.

NUTRITION DATA PER SLICE:
115 kcal (482 kJ), CHO 21g, protein 3g, fat 2g.

THE DETAILED FOOD VALUE LISTS

We have included this food value chart to help you find out more about food and what's in it. Most people use a limited range of food in their day-to-day eating pattern, but we now know that eating a wide range of foods helps to make sure we get a nutritious diet. This list may give you the confidence to include a wider variety of food when eating out, or at home.

We have given you the glycaemic index factor for individual foods where this is known and the amount of energy, carbohydrate, protein and fat in different food items. Quantities of foods have been given in 'average servings' to allow you to compare them.

The tables are based on information supplied by the Australian Department of Health and *The GI Factor* by Dr Jennie Brand Miller, Kaye Foster-Powell, Dr Stephen Colagiuri and Dr Anthony Leeds. Note that foods are generally rated as being low glycaemic index if their GI factor is below 55; intermediate glycaemic index if their GI factor is between 55 and 70; and high glycaemic index if their GI factor is more than 70. Most of the foods are roughly equivalent to those found in the UK. For specific information about UK foods, check labels or talk to your dietician.

Foods vary greatly in their nutrition content, depending on factors such as place of origin, ripeness and season. In view of this, we have rounded off all figures for nutrients to the nearest whole number and weights of foods, where appropriate, to the nearest 5g. The value of commercial products varies with brands—a reminder to read labels. Use this chart as a guide only to nutrition values. Foods have been arranged according to food groups and listed alphabetically.

NOTE: CHO = carbohydrate   Prot = protein   Alc =alcohol   neg = negligible

G.I.	FOODS	SERVING SIZE	ENERGY kJ	kcal	FAT g	CHO g	Prot g
BREAKFAST CEREALS							
42 (av.)	All-bran™	½ cup (35g)	358	85	2	13	5
55	Bran, oat, raw	1 tbsp (10g)	113	27	1	6	2
	Bran flakes	1 cup (45g)	617	147	1	28	6
77 (av.)	Coco-pops	1 cup (45g)	729	174	1	40	2
84 (av.)	Corn-flakes	1 cup (30g)	474	113	neg.	25	2
56	Muesli, unsweetened, untoasted	1 cup (65g)	888	202	6	33	8
66	Nutrigrain™	1 cup (30g)	484	116	0	20	7
	Oats, rolled, raw	⅓ cup (30g)	490	117	3	20	4
46 (av.)	Oats, rolled, cooked	1 cup (260g)	551	132	3	22	4
80	Puffed wheat	1 cup (12g)	181	43	neg.	9	2
83	Rice krispies	1 cup (30g)	444	106	neg.	24	2
54	Special-K™	1 cup (30g)	481	115	1	22	6
73	Sultana Bran™	1 cup (54g)	687	164	1	28	5
68	Sustain™	½ cup (30g)	477	114	2	32	3
74	Wheat flakes	1 cup (30g)	452	108	neg.	22	4

G.I.	FOODS	SERVING SIZE	ENERGY kJ	ENERGY kcal	FAT g	CHO g	Prot g
BREAKFAST CEREALS continued							
	Wheatgerm	2 tbsp (12g)	134	32	1	3	3
61	Wheat bisks, e.g. Weetabix™	2 bisc. (30g)	399	95	1	19	3
GRAINS AND PASTAS							
48 (av.)	Cracked wheat	¼ cup (45g)	563	134	1	27	5
	Cornflour	2 tbsp (20g)	312	75	0	18	0
65 (av.)	Couscous	⅔ cup (120g)	555	133	0	26	
43	Custard, commercial	½ cup (130g)	510	122	4	18	4
	Flour, wheat, wholemeal	½ cup (70g)	819	196		37	8
	Flour, wheat, white, plain	½ cup (70g)	1028	246	1	51	8
25 (av.)	Pearl barley	2 tbsp (35g)	446	107	1	21	32
	Pasta, white, macaroni, spaghetti, dry	100g	1430	341	1	70	11
43 (av.)	Pasta, white, macaroni, spaghetti, boiled	1 cup (180g)	696 / 895	166 / 214	0 / 1	34 / 44	6 / 7
	Pasta, egg, boiled	1 cup (200g)	1094	261	1	51	11
	Rice, brown, raw	3 tbsp (50g)	716	171	1	36	4
76	Rice, brown, boiled	1 cup (180g)	1134	271	2	57	6
	Rice, white, raw	3 tbsp (50g)	723	173	0	36	3
87	Rice, white, boiled	1 cup (190g)	994	237	0	53	4
58 (av.)	Rice, basmati	1 cup (190g)	998	237	0	55	4
	Sago, dry	2 tbsp (20g)	300	72	0	18	neg.
55	Semolina, dry	2 tbsp (25g)	346	83	0	17	3
55	Semolina, cooked	1 cup (245g)	314	75	0	15	2
68	Taco shells	3 small (33g)	693	166	9	20	2
BREADS							
69 (av.)	Bread, wholegrain	1 slice (30g)	282	67	1	12	3
76	Bread, rye, dark	1 slice (50g)	424	101	1	19	4
	Bread, white, high fibre	1 slice (28g)	272	65	1	12	3
70 (av.)	Bread, white, regular	1 slice (28g)	291	70	1	13	2
69 (av.)	Bread roll, wholemeal	1 av. (105g)	1050	251	3	46	11
70 (av.)	Bread roll, white	1 av. (190g)	972	232	2	44	9
57	Bread, pitta, white	1 large (110g)	1232	294	3	57	10
57	Bread, pitta, white	1 small (65g)	728	174	1	34	6
	Breadcrumbs, commercial	2 tbsp (14g)	213	51	1	9	2
72	Bagel	1 med. (80g)	720	179	3	32	8
69	Crumpet, regular	1 (50g)	390	93	0	20	3
67	Croissant	1 (65g)	1066	255	15	23	7
45 (av.)	Muffin, English	2 halves (80g)	669	160	1	29	8
BISCUITS							
	Crackerbread™	4 (28g)	482	115	3	19	4
	Gingernuts	2 (27g)	470	112	2	23	1

G.I.	FOODS	SERVING SIZE	ENERGY kJ	kcal	FAT g	CHO g	Prot g
BISCUITS continued							
	Krispy Wheat™, Seaswheat™	4 (20g)	384	92	3	14	2
79	Morning Coffee™	2 (16g)	290	68	2	13	1
	Marie	2 (16g)	300	70	2	13	1
69	Ryvita™	2 (20g)	301	72	1	16	2
62	Savoy™	6 (125g)	470	113	5	17	2
	Shredded Wheat™	2 (16g)	270	64	2	11	1
PULSES							
	Baked beans, canned	½ cup (120g)	324	77	1	12	6
	Chick peas, uncooked	1 tbsp (25g)	339	81	neg.	11	5
33 (av.)	Chick peas, cooked	½ cup (80g)	424	102	neg.	14	7
	Dried beans, (borlotti, haricot, white, black-eyed, etc.), uncooked	1 tbsp (25g)	290	69	neg.	10	6
40 (av.)	Dried beans, cooked	½ cup (90g)	375	84	neg.	17	6
	Lentils, uncooked	1 tbsp (25g)	352	84	neg.	15	6
26 (av.)	Lentils, cooked	½ cup (70g)	294	69	neg.	13	6
	Mixed bean salad, canned	½ cup (100g)	446	106	1	17	6
	Soya beans, raw	1 tbsp (25g)	426	102	4	9	9
14	Soya beans, canned	½ cup (100g)	466	111	4	10	11
	Split peas, raw	1 tbsp (25g)	364	87	neg.	16	6
32	Split peas, cooked	½ cup (90g)	433	103	neg.	19	7
STARCHY VEGETABLES cooked, edible portions							
85 (av.)	Potato—baked (no fat)	1 medium (120g)	343	82	0	17	3
62 (av.)	new	5 small (175g)	460	110	0	22	4
56	boiled	1 medium (120g)	313	75	0	15	3
	french fries	120g	1236	295	17	31	5
97	Parsnip, peeled, boiled	½ cup (75g)	156	37	0	8	1
55	Sweetcorn, frozen, boiled	½ cup (90g)	373	89	1	17	3
54	Sweet potato	½ cup (120g)	321	77	0	17	2
51	Yam	½ cup (120g)	473	113	0	27	3

LOW STARCH VEGETABLES

Where ½ cup cooked vegetables provides 5g or less of carbohydrate, we have classified them as 'low starch vegetables'. These vegetables are also low in calories, protein and fat, but high in vitamins, minerals and fibre. Include them in your daily meal plan.

The GI values are not determined for very low starch vegetables as their effect on blood glucose levels are negligible. Where vegetables in this list provide some starch, the GI factor is shown in brackets.

artichoke, globe	capsicum (bell pepper)	garlic	radish
asparagus	carrot (49)	kale	spinach
bean shoots/sprouts	cauliflower	lettuce	summersquash/baby squash
beans, french	celery	marrow	swede (72)
beetroot (64)	Chinese broccoli	mushrooms	tomato
bok choy	Chinese cabbage	mung beans/sprouts	turnip
broad beans (79)	courgette	onion	watercress
broccoli	cucumber	parsley	
brussel sprouts	aubergine	peas (48 av.)	
cabbage	endive	pumpkin (75)	

G.I.	FOODS	SERVING SIZE	ENERGY kJ	kcal	FAT g	CHO g	Prot g
FRUIT, edible portion							
38 (av.)	Apple, fresh	1 (155g)	323	77	0	19	0
	Apple, canned/stewed	1 cup (240g)	327	79	0	20	0
40	Apple juice, unsweetened	½ cup (125ml)	220	53	0	14	0
57	Apricot, fresh	3 medium (100g)	156	37	0	7	1
64	Apricot, canned/stewed	1 cup (230g)	228	55	0	12	2
31	Apricot, dried	5 pieces (30g)	246	59	0	13	1
	Avocado	¼ medium (75g)	659	157	17	0	1
55 (av.)	Banana	1 medium (140g)	501	120	0	28	2
	Berries, blackberry/raspberry	1 cup (135g)	140	33	0	7	1
	Berries, blueberry	1 cup (135g)	320	76	0	19	1
	Berries, strawberry	12 med. (100g)	81	19	0	3	2
22	Cherries	20 medium (80g)	179	43	0	10	1
	Date, dried	5 whole (40g)	422	101	0	25	1
	Fig, fresh	2 whole (95g)	161	30	0	8	1
	Fig, dried	2 whole (30g)	272	65	0	16	1
	Gooseberry, stewed, unsweetened	½ cup (125g)	78	19	0	4	1
25	Grapefruit, fresh	½ (120g)	133	32	0	6	1
48	Grapefruit, juice, unsweetened	½ cup (125ml)	152	36	0	8	0
46 (av.)	Grapes	1 cup (170g)	435	104	0	25	1
	Honey dew melon	¼ medium (150g)	194	46	0	10	1
52 (av.)	Kiwi fruit	1 medium (80g)	159	38	0	8	1
	Lemon	1 medium (50g)	48	12	0	2	0
	Lime	1 medium (30g)	27	6	0	1	0
	Lychee	9 whole (100g)	286	68	0	16	1
	Mandarin	1 medium (75g)	122	29	0	6	1
55 (av.)	Mango	1 small (150g)	349	83	0	19	1
	Nectarine	2 medium (100g)	156	37	0	8	1
44 (av.)	Orange	1 whole (120g)	190	45	0	10	1
46 (av.)	Orange, juice, unsweetened	125ml	178	42	0	10	1
	Passionfruit, pulp	1 medium (20g)	39	9	0	1	1
58 (av.)	Paw Paw (papaya)	1 small (200g)	246	59	0	14	1
42 (av.)	Peach, fresh	1 medium (90g)	115	27	0	6	1
30	Peach, canned, unsweetened	1 cup (210g)	353	84	0	19	2
38 (av.)	Pear, fresh	1 medium (90g)	115	27	0	6	1

G.I.	FOODS	SERVING SIZE	ENERGY kJ	kcal	FAT g	CHO g	Prot g
FRUIT, edible portion							
44	Pear, canned, unsweetened	1 cup (200g)	220	53	0	13	0
66	Pineapple, fresh	1 slice (110g)	174	42	0	9	1
46	Pineapple, juice	½ cup (125ml)	244	58	0	14	1
	Pineapple, can, unsweetened	2 slices (100g)	187	45	0	10	1
39 (av.)	Plum	1 large (100g)	155	37	0	8	1
	Prune, dried	6 medium (50g)	343	82	0	20	1
64	Raisin	¼ cup (40g)	488	117	0	28	1
56	Sultana	¼ cup (48g)	614	147	0	36	1
	Rhubarb, stewed, unsweetened	½ cup (130g)	33	8	0	1	1
65	Rock melon, canteloupe	¼ (200g)	182	43	0	9	1
72	Watermelon	1 cup (195g)	187	45	0	10	1
MILK AND DAIRY PRODUCTS							
	Cheese,						
	cottage, low-fat	½ cup (100g)	362	86	1	2	18
	block, low-fat 7%	30g	242	58	2	0	10
	ricotta, low-fat	60g	332	79	5	1	7
	block, low-fat 18%	30g	360	90	5	0	20
	cheddar	30g	504	120	10	0	8
	cream	30g	431	103	10	0	2
	cream, low-fat, 14%	10g	70	17	1	0	1
	Ice cream						
50	regular	2 scoops (48g)	384	92	5	10	2
	low-fat	2 scoops (48g)	291	70	3	9	2
	Milk,						
32	skimmed	1 cup (250ml)	369	88	0	13	9
	powder, skimmed	3 tbsp (33g)	499	119	0	17	12
	evaporated, skimmed	½ cup (162g)	689	164	0	24	17
	2% fat	1 cup (250ml)	606	145	5	15	10
27 (av.)	full cream	1 cup (250ml)	707	169	10	12	9
	powder, full cream	3 tbsp (27g)	554	132	7	11	7
	evaporated, full cream	½ cup (162g)	1069	255	15	18	14
31	So Good, soy milk	1 cup (250ml)	650	155	9	12	9
	Yoghurt,						
14	low-fat, natural	1 tub (200g)	420	110	0	13	12
33	wholemilk,, natural	1 tub (200g)	650	155	8	13	9
	diet	1 tub (200g)	380	90	0	13	9
	low-fat flavoured/fruit	1 tub (200g)	744	178	2	32	10
61	wholemilk, flavoured/fruit	1 tub (200g)	826	197	4	32	10
PROTEIN FOODS							
	Egg, hen	1 medium (55g)	288	69	0	9	6
	Fish and seafood,						
	fish, raw	1 fillet (100g)	386	92	2	0	18
	oysters, raw	½ dozen (60g)	130	31	1	0	6

G.I.	FOODS	SERVING SIZE	ENERGY kJ	kcal	FAT g	CHO g	Prot g
PROTEIN FOODS							
	prawns, boiled	100g	451	108	2	0	22
	tuna/salmon, canned in brine, drained	½ cup (90g)	411	98	2	0	20
38	fish fingers, oven cooked	5 (125g)	1175	281	14	24	15
	Meat and meat products,						
	beef, lean, minced	120g	581	139	4	0	26
	beef, raw, lean only	120g	602	144	4	0	26
	ham, leg, lean	1 slice (30g)	136	32	1	0	6
	lamb, raw, lean only	120g	608	145	4	0	26
	liver	120g	816	195	9	3	26
	luncheon meat	1 slice (30g)	321	77	6	1	4
28	pork, raw, lean only	120g	531	127	2	0	27
	pork sausage, fried	2 (75g)	818	195	15	4	12
	salami	3 slices (30g)	538	128	11	0	7
	veal, raw, lean only	20g	531	127	2	0	27
	Nuts,						
	almonds, raw	⅓ cup (50g)	1168	278	27	2	5
	peanuts, raw	⅓ cup (50g)	1182	281	25	5	12
	pecans, raw	⅓ cup, 50g	1379	328	36	2	5
	walnuts, raw	⅓ cup (50g)	1425	340	35	2	7
	pine nuts, raw	20g	498	119	11	3	4
	peanut butter	1 tbsp (20g)	516	123	11	2	5
	Poultry,						
	chicken, breast, no skin, raw	120g	563	135	3	0	27
	Tofu/soy bean curd	½ cup (110g)	303	72	6	2	8
FATS AND HIGH SNACK FOODS							
	Cream, thickened	2 tbsp (40g)	547	131	14	1	1
	Corn chips	50g	990	237	13	25	4
	Dressing, french	2 tbsp (40g)	625	149	16	3	0
	Mayonnaise, reduced-fat	1 tbsp (20g)	258	62	5	3	0
	Margarine/butter	1 tbsp (20g)	608	145	16	0	0
	Olives, in brine	4 medium (27g)	113	27	3	0	0
	Oil	1 tbsp	702	168	19	0	0
54 (av.)	Potato crisps, plain	50g	1050	251	16	24	3
	Popcorn, plain	20g	392	94	5	11	2
SUGARS, CONFECTIONERY AND MISCELLANEOUS							
49	Chocolate, milk	6 squares (30g)	645	154	8	19	2
66	Cordial, diluted	1 cup (250ml)	355	85	0	20	0
23 (av.)	Fructose	10g	167	40	0	10	0
100	Glucose	10g	167	40	0	10	0
58	Honey	1 tbsp (20g)	264	63	0	16	0
80	Jelly beans	15g	170	40	0	10	1
46 (av.)	Lactose	10g	167	40	0	10	0

G.I.	FOODS	SERVING SIZE	ENERGY kJ	kcal	FAT g	CHO g	Prot g
	SUGARS, CONFECTIONERY AND MISCELLANEOUS continued						
68	Mars Bar™	1 bar (63g)	1090	260	11	39	3
61	Muesli Bar, fruit	1 bar (31g)	481	115	5	17	1
65 (av.)	Sucrose	2 tsp (10g)	167	40	0	10	0
68	Soft drink	1 can (375ml)	829	198	0	51	0

ALCOHOLIC BEVERAGES

1 standard drink = approximately 10g alcohol and 80 calories (335 kJ) with the exception of alcohol-reduced drinks.

FOODS	SERVING ml	ENERGY kJ	kcal	CHO g	Alc g
Beer,					
low alcohol beer	200	87	21	2	1
light beer, 2–3% alcohol	200	190–250	46–60	4–6	4–6
ordinary beer, 3.5–4% alcohol	200	300–335	72–80	4–6	7–8
CHO modified 'diet' beer	200	250	60	2	7
stout	200	462	110	6	12
Wine,					
white, dry	120	340	80	neg.	12
red, dry	120	340	80	neg.	12
champagne, dry	120	340	80	neg. –2	12
white, sweet	120	335	80	3–4	9–10
Other,					
spirits, brandy, gin, rum, whisky	30	276	66	0	10
sherry, dry	60	335	80	1	9
sherry, sweet	60	365	90	4	11
vermouth, dry	60	335	80	1	11
vermouth, sweet	60	365	90	4	11
cider	200	335	80	2	10
liqueurs	20	300	70	6	7
port	60	260	60	8	10

INDEX